THE WORLD OF
HAIR COLOUR

A Scientific Companion

HAIRDRESSING

Mahogany Hairdressing: Steps to Cutting, Colouring and Finishing Hair
Martin Gannon and Richard Thompson

Mahogany Hairdressing: Advanced Looks *Richard Thompson and Martin Gannon*

Essensuals, Next Generation Toni & Guy: Step by Step

Professional Men's Hairdressing *Guy Kremer and Jacki Wadeson*

The Art of Dressing Long Hair *Guy Kremer and Jacki Wadeson*

Patrick Cameron: Dressing Long Hair *Patrick Cameron and Jacki Wadeson*

Patrick Cameron: Dressing Long Hair Book 2 *Patrick Cameron*

Bridal Hair *Pat Dixon and Jacki Wadeson*

Trevor Sorbie: Visions in Hair *Kris Sorbie and Jacki Wadeson*

The Total Look: The Style Guide for Hair and Make-up Professionals *Ian Mistlin*

Art of Hair Colouring *David Adams and Jacki Wadeson*

Begin Hairdressing: The Official Guide to Level 1 *Martin Green*

Hairdressing – The Foundations: The Official Guide to Level 2
Leo Palladino (contribution Jane Farr)

Professional Hairdressing: The Official Guide to Level 3 4e *Martin Green, Lesley Kimber
and Leo Palladino*

Men's Hairdressing: Traditional and Modern Barbering 2e *Maurice Lister*

African-Caribbean Hairdressing 2e *Sandra Gittens*

Salon Management *Martin Green*

eXtensions: The Official Guide to Hair Extensions *Theresa Bullock*

BEAUTY THERAPY

Beauty Therapy – The Foundations: The Official Guide to Level 2 *Lorraine Nordmann*

Beauty Basics – The Official Guide to Level 1 *Lorraine Nordmann*

Professional Beauty Therapy: The Official Guide to Level 3 *Lorraine Nordmann,
Lorraine Williamson, Jo Crowder and Pamela Linforth*

Aromatherapy for the Beauty Therapist *Valerie Ann Worwood*

Indian Head Massage *Muriel Burnham-Airey and Adele O'Keefe*

The Official Guide to Body Massage *Adele O'Keefe*

An Holistic Guide to Anatomy and Physiology *Tina Parsons*

The Encyclopedia of Nails *Jacqui Jefford and Anne Swain*

Nail Artistry *Jacqui Jefford, Sue Marsh and Anne Swain*

The Complete Nail Technician *Marian Newman*

The World of Skin Care: A Scientific Companion *Dr John Gray*

Safety in the Salon *Elaine Almond*

An Holistic Guide to Reflexology *Tina Parsons*

Nutrition: A Practical Approach *Suzanne Le Quesne*

An Holistic Guide to Massage *Tina Parsons*

THE WORLD OF
HAIR COLOUR

A Scientific Companion

Dr JOHN GRAY

Sponsors

P&Gbeauty

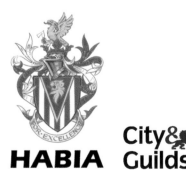

HABIA   City&Guilds   **THOMSON**

Australia • Canada • Mexico • Singapore • Spain • United Kingdom • United States

THOMSON

The World of Hair Colour: A Scientific Companion

Copyright © 2005 Dr John Gray

The Thomson logo is a registered trademark used herein under licence.

For more information, contact Thomson Learning, High Holborn House, 50–51 Bedford Row, London WC1R 4LR or visit us on the World Wide Web at: http://www.thomsonlearning.co.uk

British Library Cataloguing-in-Publication Data
A catalogue record for this book is available from the British Library

ISBN 1-84480-043-1

First edition published 2005 by Thomson Learning

Typeset by 🅣 Tek-Art, Croydon, Surrey
Printed in Croatia by Zrinski d.d.

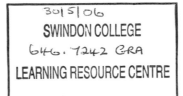

'Colour; above all ... is a means of liberation ... the freeing of conventions'
Henri Matisse

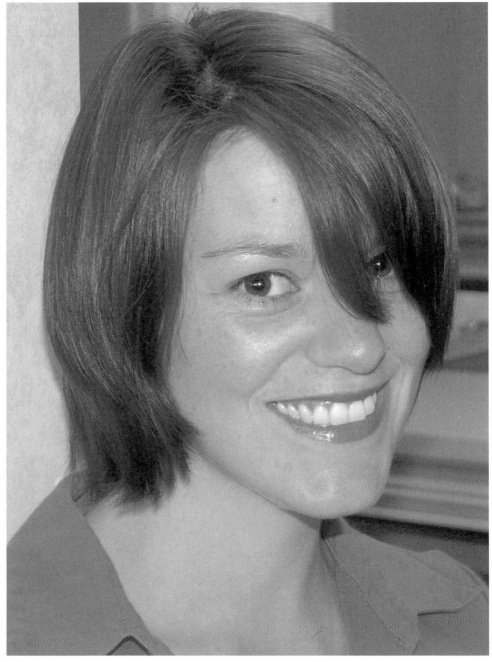

Red – worldwide the most frequent artificial hair colour, here seen to perfection.

'Hair colour – a must becomes a lust'
Carola Wacker – Meister Wella

'Hair colour – a change is often to deceive'
William Shakespeare, *Henry IV*

Contents

Introduction   1

1. Colour in the world   3

2. Human hair colour   7
Human hair function   8
Modern humans and hair colour   8
Colour, sight and evolution   12
Colour and the human eye   12
Hair colour and the human eye   13
Interpretation of colour   14
Colour terminology   16
Colour systems   17

3. Hair pigments and the hair follicle   19
Hair colour pigments   19
Hair colour from the follicle to the tip   21
Pigmentation from youth to old age   26
Hair colour   28
Loss of hair pigments   29
Weathering   29
Grey hair   30

4. Human hair colour in history   37
Hair colour and its social implications   37
Black, brunette, red and blonde   43

5. Hair colour products   51
Artificial hair colour throughout history   53
Modern hair dyes   57
Permanent hair dyeing   67
The colour transformation   72
How to choose the right shade   77
Natural and vegetable colouring agents   78

6. **Colouring hair: scientific and practical aspects**   **81**
   Actual on-head colours   81
   Classical palette   85
   Step-by-step colouring   86
   Roots   91

7. **Tips from the experts**   **93**
   Going blonde   93
   Practical steps in going blonde   94
   Going red   100
   Going brunette   100
   Covering the grey   100
   Caring for your colour   104
   Colour problems   105

8. **The safety of hair dyes**   **111**

9. **Hair colour products: regulatory issues**   **115**
   Worldwide regulations   115
   European regulations   116
   US regulations   116
   Japanese regulations   117
   Some regulatory considerations for other countries   117

   Index   119

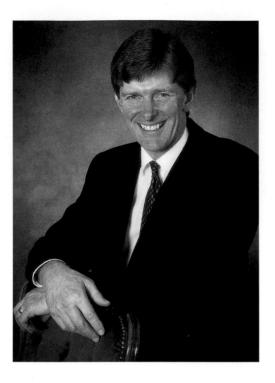

The author

John Gray received his medical degree from St George's Hospital London, and is a family practitioner and a practising trichologist in the UK. He is Medical Adviser to Procter & Gamble Beauty.

Dr Gray is a member of the European and North American Hair Research Societies and of the European Society of Contact Dermatitis, and has been elected to the Royal Society of Medicine. He is also a member of the Institute of Trichologists. He has written two other books in the 'World of…' series, *The World of Hair* and *The World of Skin Care*, in addition to *Human Hair Diversity, A Pocket Book of Hair Disorders* (in collaboration with Dr R Dawber) and *Dandruff – Aetiology, Pathophysiology and Treatment*, and many other chapters and publications on hair.

He is an Executive Director of the Oxford Hair Foundation, and has recently broadcast on BBC4 and the BBC World Service on hair and its problems. He has just been appointed Associate Editor of the *International Journal of Cosmetic Dermatology*.

The contributors

Dr Chris Gummer
Leading hair scientist with Procter & Gamble Beauty Care, Europe, and board member of the Oxford Hair Foundation. After gaining his doctorate at Oxford in genetic hair diseases and hair ultrastructure, he moved to the University Medical School, San Francisco, CA to study transdermal drug delivery. He joined Richardson Vicks and then Procter & Gamble in 1985. Numerous publications and presentations in both fundamental biology and cosmetic science along with industry awards mean that he is now recognized as a world leading authority on hair and skin cosmetic science. He received a top industry accolade from the Society of Cosmetic Chemists, who awarded him The Joseph P. Ciaudelli award for 'best scientific paper of 2002' for his paper entitled 'Elucidating penetration pathways into the hair fibre using novel microscopic techniques'. This publication revealed the mechanisms whereby complex molecules penetrate the hair shaft prior to creating colour.

Dr Elizabeth Desmond
Principal Scientist, Procter & Gamble Beauty Care, Europe. Elizabeth Desmond has a BSc Hons in microbiology from University College Cork, Ireland and a PhD in molecular biology from the University of Reading, UK. She joined Procter & Gamble Beauty Care Research and Development in 1996, and since 1998 has specialized in upstream hair colour research. Her world-class expertise is in detailed consumer research to understand the key needs of the colorant consumer. She is currently responsible for the western Europe, Middle East and African Clairol hair colour markets.

Dr Steven Shiel
After gaining a first-class chemistry degree from University College Swansea he obtained the DESU diploma from the Ecole Nationale Supérieure de Chimie de Montpellier and a PhD in organometallic chemistry from the University of Birmingham. Joining P&G in 1997 in product research, he is now Scientific Communications Manager for Hair Care in Western Europe, responsible for diffusion of technical materials, and has a profound knowledge of hair care products.

Dr Jennifer Marsh
After gaining her chemistry degree at Magdalen College, Oxford and a PhD in inorganic chemistry at Wolfson College, Oxford, she did two years post-doctoral studies at Texas A&M University. She joined Procter & Gamble in 1995, and has worked in the field of hair colour for five years. She is now a Principal Scientist with Procter & Gamble Beauty Care, Europe, and is regarded as one of the leading research scientists in the field of hair colour technology.

Dr Raniero DeStasio
Raniero DeStasio has an MSc in biology and molecular virology from the University of Rome, and a PhD in microbiology and virology from Indiana University, USA. He joined Procter & Gamble in 1989 and is an Associate Director in Regulatory and Safety with involvement in the design of most of the marketed P&G beauty products including hair dyes. His key mission is ensuring that technical and science questions and issues are correctly addressed. He defines himself as a 'technical crystal ball' manager.

Foreword

Take a moment to think about the significance of colour in your life. How colour affects you, how colour may change your perception and the impact colour has in hairdressing. Colour is an integral part of the experience of visiting a salon. The correct use of colour can really compliment and dazzle a spectacular haircut and transform a client's appearance.

Dr John Gray is a practicing GP and professional trichologist who is fascinated by the hair and scalp and lends his talents and scientific expertise to writing books. Author of the successful *World of …Series*, first *The World of Hair* followed by *The World of Skin Care*, it is rewarding to see Dr John Gray lend his scientific expertise and knowledge to the complex world of hair colour and produce another text to add to the *World of* series.

Dr John Gray's enthusiasm for his subject knows no bounds. For any scientific knowledge you need to know about the hair and scalp and to really understand the science of hair colour here is a wonderful opportunity.

Alan Goldsbro
CEO HABIA

The following is an extract of a speech at Oxford Hair Foundation Seminar London, 14 November 2003 by DR CHRIS GUMMER, *Procter & Gamble*.

The ability to change hair colour with temporary or permanent dyes almost at a moment's notice brings tremendous personal power. Whether we are aiming to hide the march of time, conforming to some peer pressure or moving with the latest trend, hair colorants allow us to override our genes, which if left to themselves would be a poor component of our fashion armamentarium.

Changing hair colour in the 21st century is more complex and challenging than ever before. Breakthroughs in hair dye chemistry are leading the way to provide a unique blend of fabulous colours and quality hair as and when we desire. Individuals can then challenge and defy stereotypes.

Acknowledgments

To my dear, and long suffering friend and editor, Jean Macqueen without whom none of this would have been possible.

I would also like to thank Kathy Phillips of *Vogue,* for permission to quote from her book *The Vogue Book of Blondes* and her inspiration for this task.

Thanks to all the contributors at P&G – I stand in awe of their knowledge and passion to bring excellence to hair colour products.

My thanks to P&G Beauty for sponsoring this work and to Clairol and Wella for their support.

Profound thanks to Professor Vera Rogiers, Vice Chair SCCP for her review of the Safety of Hair Dyes and support for this publication.

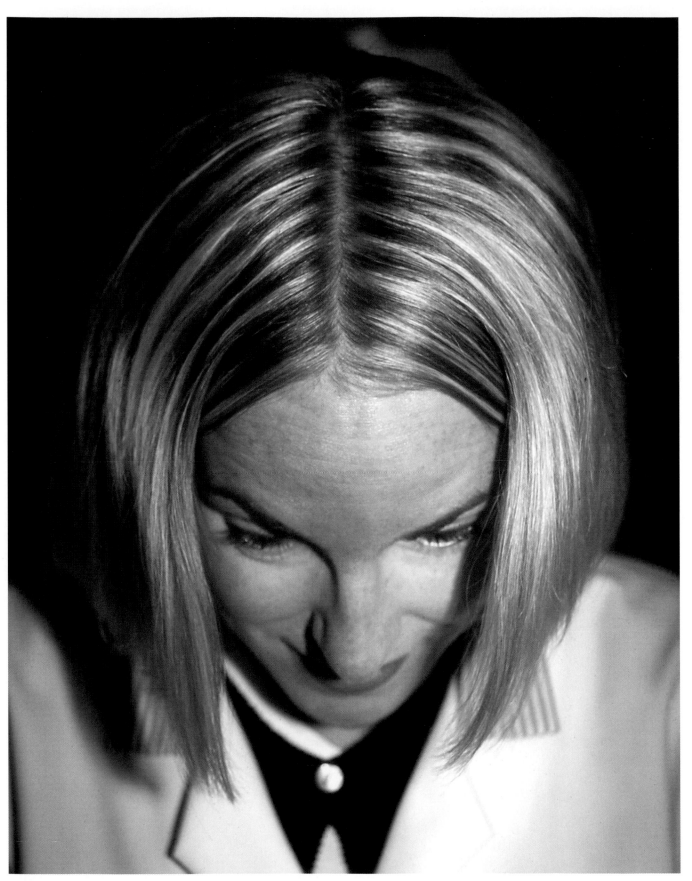

Highlights the professional way.

Introduction

This book in the 'World of ...' series is about hair colour, both natural and artificial.

Why is hair colour so important, and why, each day, do millions of women (and men) around the world feel the need to use hair dye products? The question needs to be seen in the context of our continuing obsession with appearance and a desire, evident throughout history, to conjure up a 'hair colour transformation'.

This book is dedicated to the scientists who have uncovered the secrets of human hair pigmentation, those whose skill and expertise have developed home and professional hair dye products and the stylists and technicians who create such wonders in the salon.

My remit was to produce a science companion on hair colour. I have tried to turn a complex science (which has everyday applications) into a readable journey.

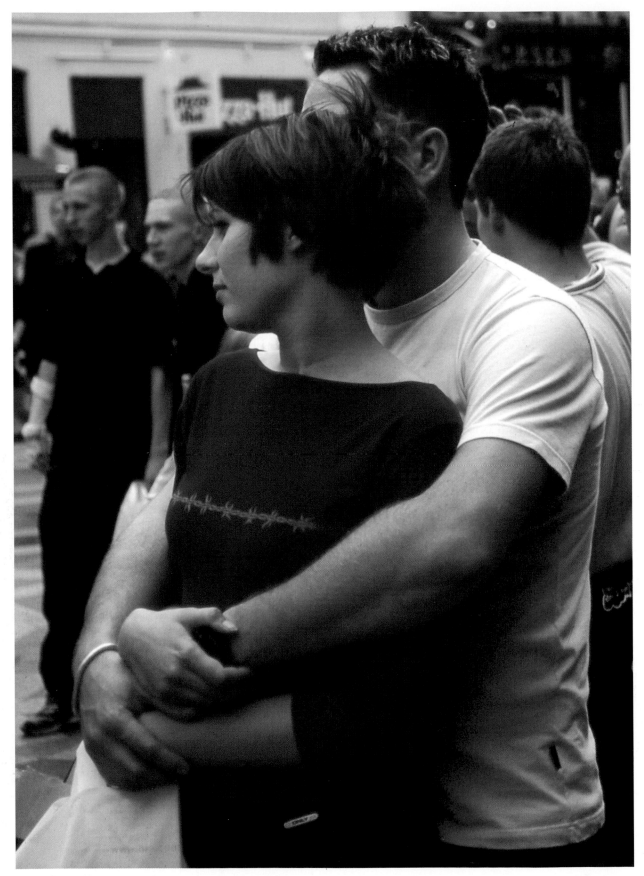

The colour of love.

1 Colour in the world

Our world is full of colour. We take for granted the blues of sky and sea, the green of grasslands and forests and the myriad glowing colours of the plant and animal kingdoms.

What then is the significance of colour in nature? Why is the world not in black and white? The answer, in part, is the source of all life – the sun. All forms of life, directly or indirectly, owe their energy and colour to sunlight.

Each species of plant and animal, from the humblest to the most elevated, has developed body colour in its evolutionary battle for a place in a light-filled world. Leaves, petals, scales, feather, fur, skin and hair have all developed colour in response to two supreme pressures: survival and mating success.

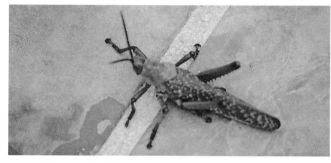

… and of the animal kingdom.

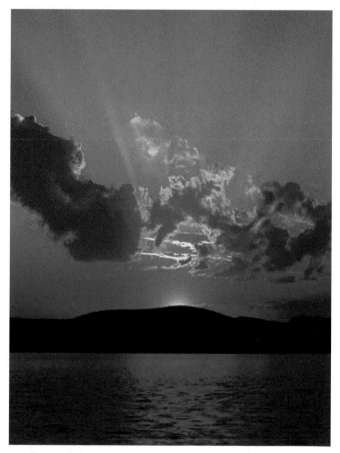

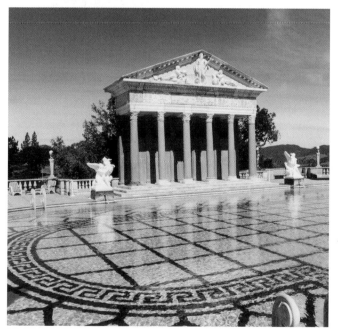

The colours of the world…

… all owe their existence to sunlight.

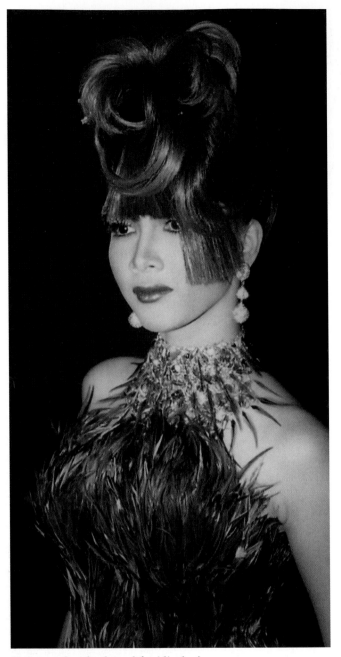

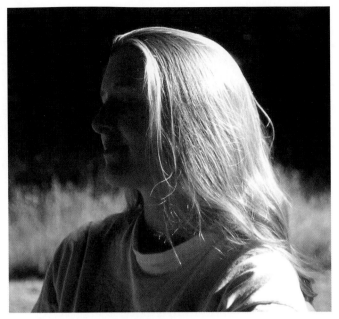

Hair is a powerful visual signal…

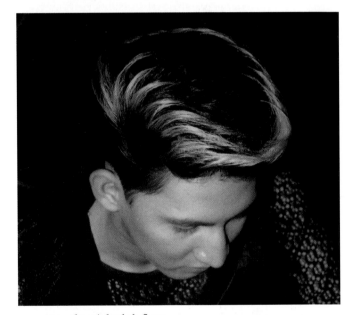

Hair – real and coloured for 'display'.

… across the nightclub floor.

From the depths of the ocean to the tops of the mountains, external body colour is a key part of individual survival, sexual attraction and perpetuation of the species. In this respect we humans are no different from other species.

All mammals, including the human species, are covered in hair, although human hair is now almost a vestigial remnant after millions of years of evolution. Emerging from equatorial forests on to the plains of Africa only six million years ago, early humans lost most (but not all) of their dense (and probably dark) body hair until it was largely confined to the scalp and sexual areas.

The functions of hair and its colour are confined primarily to recognition and display at a distance, denoting age, sex, ethnic origin and, by contrivance, social position. Across the open plain or the nightclub floor, hair is the most powerful visual signal of attraction (or repellence).

The male peacock that must win but a single mate exhibits the most outrageous signal to do so. *Homo sapiens* sometimes mimic this display with the same (and sometimes forlorn) hope.

The broad stripe of the silverback male gorilla is associated with sexual attraction and dominance. We might argue that the same is true

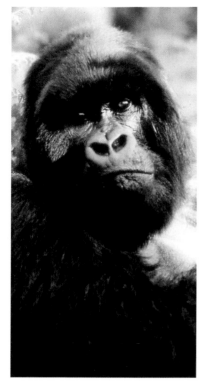

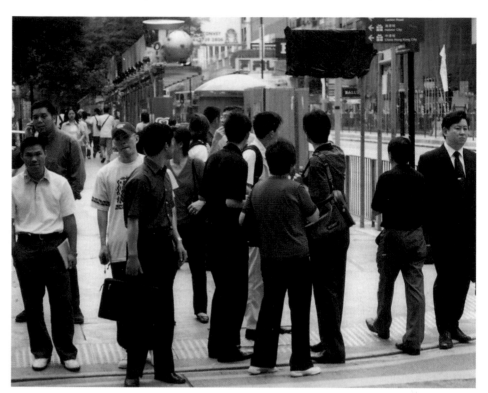

Most primates…   *and humans have black hair…*

in *Homo sapiens*, where a crown of white hair is often synonymous with status and power.

Hair colour, as well as hair form, is determined by the combination of genes donated by our parents, and often reflects our wider family, lineage and descent.

Although black hair is the dominant colour of humankind, in our short recorded history the desire to change one's natural colour, whether for personal, social or cultural reasons, is self-evident.

Hair colour is one of the strongest communication 'strategies' we have and is capable of influencing others in many and subtle ways (Dr Linda Papadopoulos). Shakespeare's King Henry IV remarked that a change of colour is 'often to deceive'. The question is, who are we attempting to deceive – ourselves or others, and why?

This book sets out to explore the World of Hair Colour – the role of our genes in determining the colour of our hair, why dark hair dominates, why naturally blonde hair is so rarely seen and why so many people are trying to go blonde.

We examine the alchemy of ancient and modern hair colour products and the benefits that hair colour transformation now brings to the quality of life of millions of women (and men).

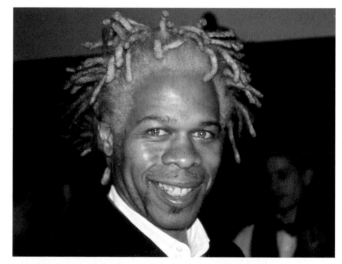

but the desire to change hair colour is widespread.

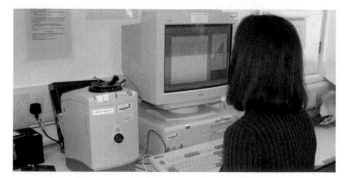

… aided by the hair alchemist of today, at work in the laboratory.

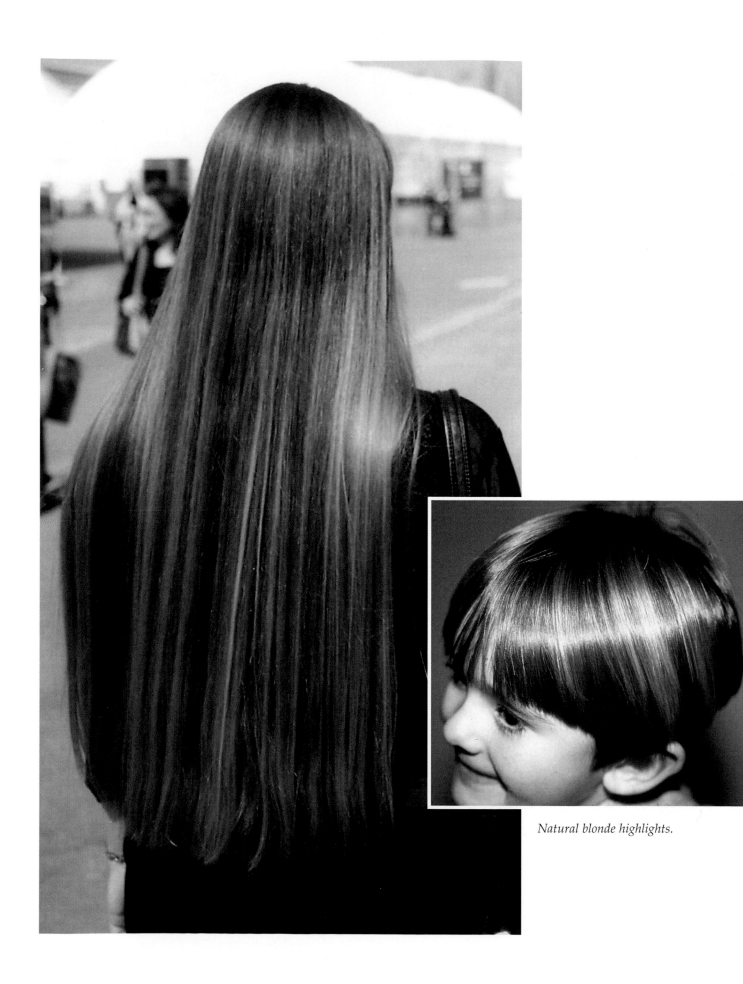

Natural blonde highlights.

Human hair colour

Human hair is our species' supreme ornamentation, capable of demonstrating ethnic origin, sex, age, personality or professional grouping.

The production of the pigments that give us our natural hair colour is under genetic control. These pigments, called **melanins**, are found in the skin, the hair follicle and the hair shaft. Melanins are responsible for most of the hair colour we see: the physical aspects of the hair fibre (shape and density) act only as minor modifiers of colour.

Curiously, and as a result of evolutionary forces, the variety of human hair colour is very limited: not for us the vivid purples and greens of the bird kingdom or the lurid phosphorescence of the fish world.

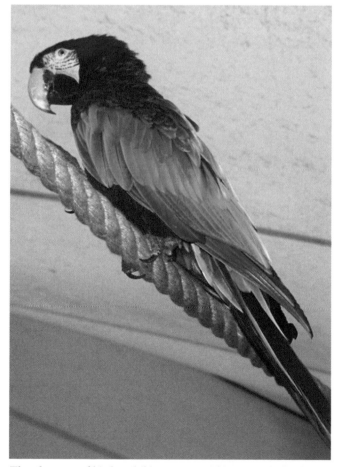

The plumage of birds exhibits an astonishing range of colour.

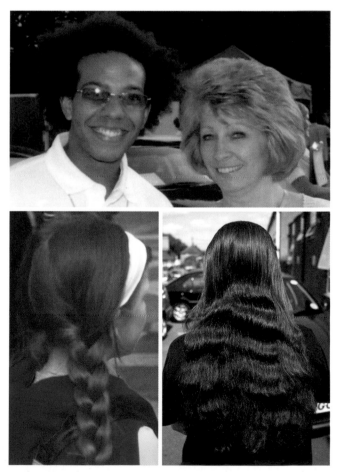

… but human hair has a more limited range.

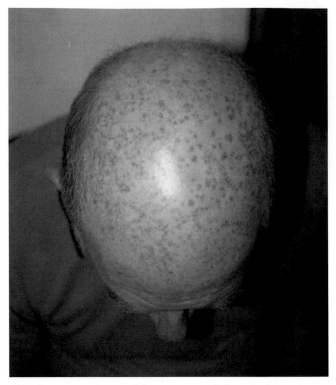

Skin damage, and even skin cancer, can follow the loss of photoprotective pigmented hair.

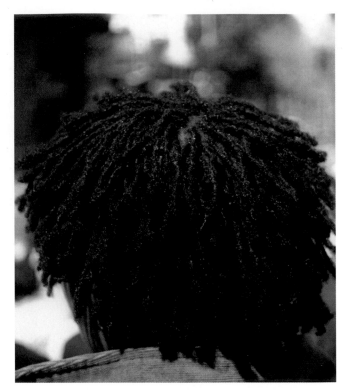

Dark hair for camouflage, insulation – and detoxification?

Human hair function

The specific function of human hair colour is still open to speculation.

Animals have clearly developed hair for camouflage, insulation, scent dispersal and mate identification.

Among many theories on human hair colour selection is the suggestion of one of the world's leading experts Dr Desmond Tobin and his colleagues that ancient human dependency on fish, which concentrate toxic heavy metals, forced evolution to a mechanism wherein darkly pigmented hair became part of a biochemical process designed to maximize excretion of these potentially harmful materials.

The view that hair is now only retained for sexual signalling has a good deal of support but in the view of the author, hair in equatorial regions serves an important thermoregulatory and photoprotective function. In Africa the retention of hair into the fifth and sixth decades of life is commonplace, and the delay in greying is suggestive of this preserved ancestral function. Loss of hair and its photoprotection leads to marked skin damage and a rising incidence of skin cancer on the exposed scalp.

Modern humans and hair colour

Modern humans almost certainly evolved in East Africa as recently as 200 000–150 000 years ago, our hominid ancestors having split from a common evolutionary line with our relatives, the 'old-world' great apes, some 6 000 000 years before.

Homo sapiens' nearest primate relatives (with whom we share 99% of our genetic material) are the bonobos, which have straight black hair covering most of the body. Interestingly, like us they experience thinning and greying of scalp and body hair as they age, together with significant frontal hair loss.

An interesting exception to the generally dark hair of primates is the deep red of the orangutang, a species that split from the common tree some time before the other apes.

Humans were probably on the verge of extinction some 100 000 years ago, as a result of climate change and other environmental pressures. Having clung on to a precarious existence, a pitiful handful of survivors left Africa some 90 000 years ago and slowly migrated along the edge of the Arabian peninsula, at a time when sea levels were much lower, into what is now south-east Asia. Asia was populated some 70 000 years ago, and

Hair colour and the recent past

- The USA and certain South American countries saw the largest influxes of these peoples, whose genetic characteristics covered the widest possible range. These are now the world's greatest genetic 'melting pots'.

- The development of hair colour diversity has increased and accelerated during this great mixing of genes, particularly in the Americas.

- Black hair still dominates in the world.

- Brunettes are common in Mid Europe/ America.

- Blondes and red are a rarity in numerical terms.

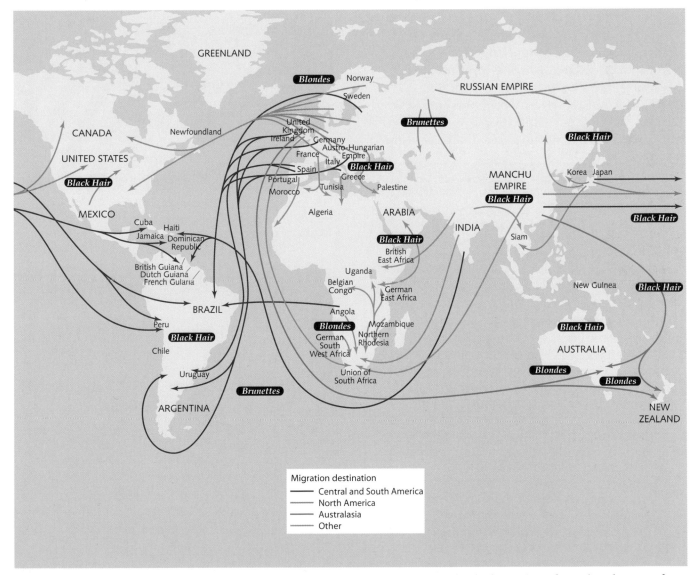

The human diaspora continues: how the varying human populations, each with its individual genetic pool, continued to spread over the world in the 19th and early 20th centuries.

[*Source* Redrawn from Blackwells, Human Hair Diversity]

Australasia 60–40 000 years ago. Europe was reached only around 35 000 years ago and the Americas much later – some 14–12 000 years ago, when humans crossed the Bering straits.

It is the genes of this early group that have been carried out into the world and proliferated, and which still dictate very largely the coloration of the now six billion inhabitants of our planet.

We can only speculate on the colour of skin and hair of the earliest modern humans, but it is highly probable that their skin was significantly pigmented for protection against equatorial levels of ultra-violet exposure. People with light skins have much less protection, and albinos in Africa invariably suffer miserably and perish with multiple skin cancers at a relatively young age even with skin protection.

It was the slow exodus of a painfully few human beings out of Africa some 100 000 years ago which took the dark hair pigment, so necessary for protection against the sun, out into the world. Only much later, probably 30–40 000 years ago, did those very few individuals who carried the gene(s) that allow lighter skin and hair colour emerge in any great numbers once out of the glare of Africa's sun.

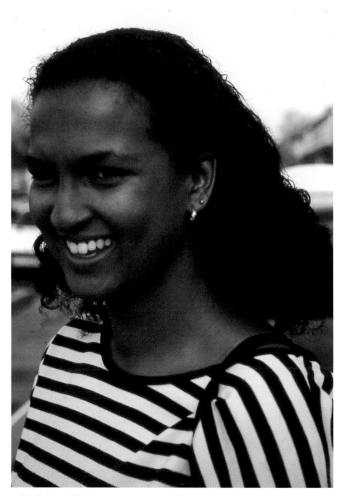

This beautiful woman has hair form and colour as close as we can tell to those of our original common mother in Africa 150 000 years ago.

SCIENCE BOX

Recent archaeological findings, by Professor Alan Cooper in Oxford, suggest that the prevalent conditions in these equatorial regions gave preferential exploitation of tiny numbers of humans favouring a body type (phenotype) best suited to flourish.

The Andamanese islanders, long regarded as an ancient African tribe left stranded on remote islands in the Indian Ocean, are in fact direct descendants of a much later Asian people. The conditions dictated that people with very darkly pigmented skins, tight curly black hair and short body stature would flourish, and under a mechanism called 'convergence' the Asian genes expression led to peoples who looked more like the much more distantly related Africans.

Early hair colour was probably equally dark but whether the tight curls of modern Africa were the original hair form is now highly debatable.

This supports the view that rapid evolutionary change or gene survival in the early groups of peoples laid the foundations for our appearance for the millennia to come.

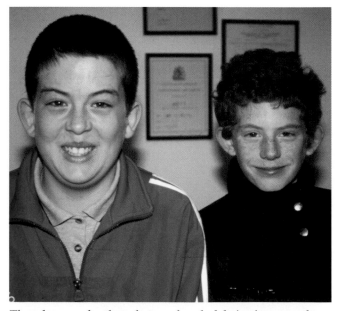

These boys are brothers, but one has dark hair pigments, the other red – even though their skin tones are similar.

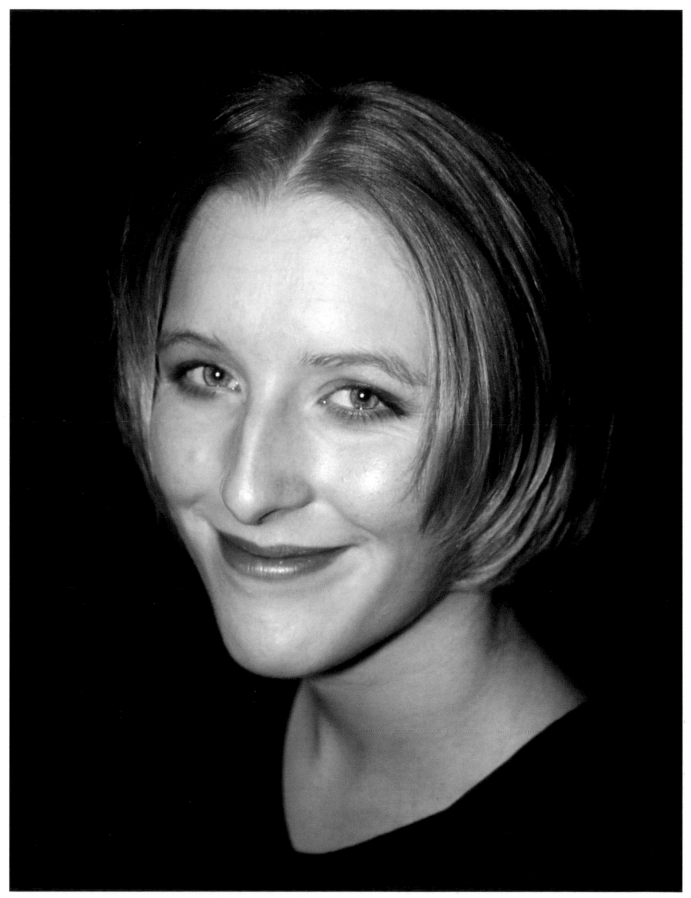

North western European natural blonde hair – a rarity in the world.

Colour, sight and evolution

Inextricably linked with the development of colour in all animal species is the specific ability to perceive it. Inevitably, both relate to the ecological niche being occupied and the prey on which that species depends for survival or protection.

On the savannahs of Africa, the zebra hides in the 'dazzle' of the herd. The adult cheetah's spots scatter light in the eyes of its prey, and may reduce the risk to cheetah cubs as they hide from other predators. The polar bear's dense white pelt, which is both thermally efficient and camouflaging, hides a dark skin.

Humans, like birds, employ almost exclusively visual signals for sexual attraction, while for many other animals – from moths to dogs – scent is the prime communication vehicle. Only those plants or animals surviving in the dark at the very bottom of the oceans or deepest caves have abandoned colour.

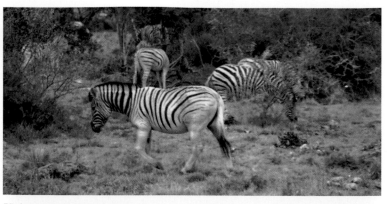

Hair patterns can deceive the eyes of a predator…

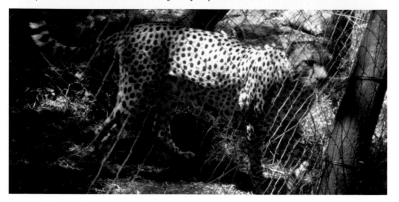

… and help to hide the predator from its prey.

SCIENCE BOX

Human beings can 'see' in three basic (primary) colours – red, yellow and blue. All other colours are based on combinations of these. People with normal colour vision can discriminate some 150 different shades.

By contrast certain species of fish have the ability to see in seven primary colours, birds four but dogs only two. The humble bee has extraordinary colour vision in order to detect its target flowers. Some birds see into the ultra-violet range, and plants that rely on these species for their pollination exploit this ability to attract them by displaying in ultra-violet 'shades'.

The chameleon can control its body colour, and, in response to seasonal sexual hormonal changes, its change of body colour indicates a desire to breed. In the primates certain mandrills and baboons retain colour variability in their posterior as a sexual signal. We humans are not at the bottom, but certainly not at the top, of the evolutionary colour tree.

Colour and the human eye

Human perception of colour in the universe is derived from the white light of the Sun.

The actual colours we 'see' are dependent on the ability of our eyes and our brains to detect and interpret the reflection of light from the world around us. Isaac Newton described in 1667 how white light can be split into its constituents in the visible range 360 nm to 830 nm.

Genetic studies indicate that our ancient ancestors in the African forests carried with them a method of discriminating different hues in the red–green range of the spectrum. Their eyes had an enhanced ability to detect colour differences by virtue of possessing three types of 'cone cells' in their retinas (see below). This was in contrast to animals that had evolved for a purely nocturnal existence, which usually have a mere single type of cone, and our eventual domestic companions, dogs, cats and cattle, which have only two.

This third type of cone cell would have been of great advantage in identifying different fruits

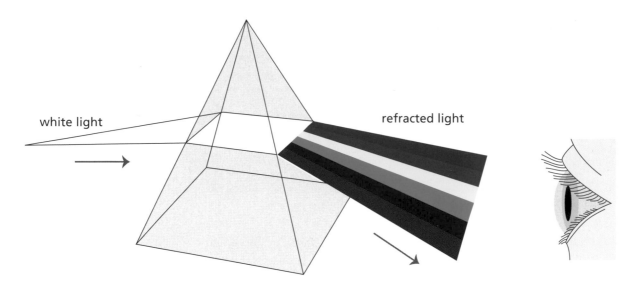

The differential refraction of light of different wavelengths as it passes through a prism (or raindrop).

and berries and for these early 'gatherers' would have endowed an evolutionary advantage. This so-called **trichromic** ability has been carried forward into modern humans.

Hair colour and the human eye

The human eye has two types of receptor (i.e. specialized sensory nerve endings) for light, both situated in the retina. Light is reflected into the eyes by objects within the so-called **visual field**. White light is a combination of *all* the colours in the visible spectrum. This is seen when light passes through a prism, which separates light of different colours by refracting (bending) the rays to different extents depending on their wavelength. Red light has the longest wavelength in the visible spectrum and violet the shortest. This differential refraction is classically seen in a rainbow.

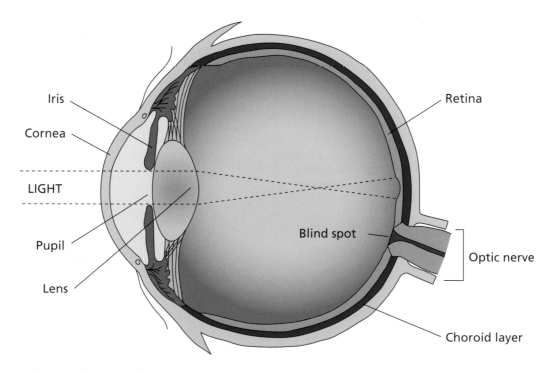

Section through the human eye.

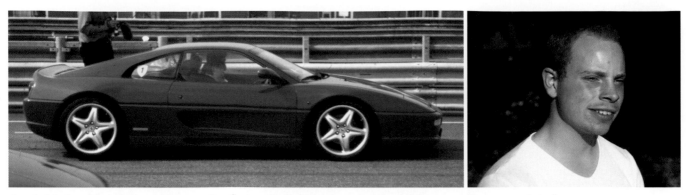

A red object and hair looks red because it reflects only light in the red region of the spectrum.

Temporary hair dye.

Beyond the highest visible wavelengths are infra-red rays, and beyond the shortest are the ultra-violet.

A specific 'pure' colour is perceived when only light of a single wavelength is reflected by the object and all the others are absorbed; for example, a red object looks red because it reflects only light in the red region of the spectrum. Objects appear white when all wavelengths are reflected, and black when they are all absorbed.

The **retina** is the photosensitive part of the eye. It contains specific nerve endings called **rods** and **cones**.

Light rays cause chemical changes in photosensitive pigments in these cells, which in their turn generate nerve impulses. These are then conducted to the brain for interpretation.

Cones are sensitive to bright light and colour. They serve vision at high levels of illumination and use a photosensitive chemical called **iodopsin**, which is only activated by bright light. In normal daylight it is these 'colour-determining' cells that are active.

There are three types of cone, described for conciseness as follows (the descriptors do not refer to the shapes of the cells):

- short, having maximum sensitivity in the short-wave (blue) region of the spectrum
- medium, with maximum sensitivity in the green region
- long, with maximum sensitivity in the red region.

Rods are more sensitive than cones, and serve vision in low light by use of a chemical (**rhodopsin**) which is monochromatic and commonly known as 'visual purple'. It is completely bleached by bright light but regenerated in the presence of adequate vitamin A. This explains the common experience that moving from bright sunshine to darkness often leads to temporary blindness – and also to the legend that carrots (rich in vitamin A) are good for night vision.

Interpretation of colour

Colour vision can be explained by perception in two stages:

- response of the three types of cone (red-, blue- and green-sensitive)
- interpretation of the stimuli by the brain.

Because the cones are sensitive to a range of wavelengths, rather than a single wavelength, overlaps occur. These similarly overlap with the

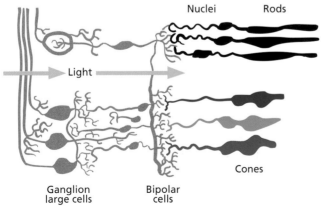

Diagrammatic section through the retina, showing the cells concerned with vision.

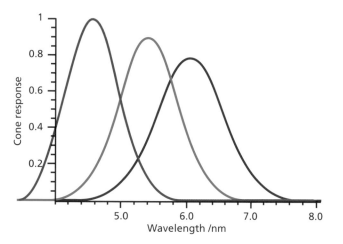

Cone cell response functions.

brain's processing (the so-called 'opponent theory') and the additive nature of light allows the full colour spectrum (plus black and white) to be seen.

Additive colour mixing

Additive colour mixing describes how the primary colours can combine to produce many other shades.

The most familiar analogy is the manner in which a television set works. A TV has only three light sources (red, green and blue), which are used at different intensities to give the image.

Light mixing is additive: for example,

Yellow = Green + Red

Mixing light of three colours (of differing wavelengths) allows large parts of the colour spectrum to be achieved. Mixing monochromatic

Red – 700.0 nm
Green – 546.1 nm
Blue – 435.8 nm

will give the maximum possible range.

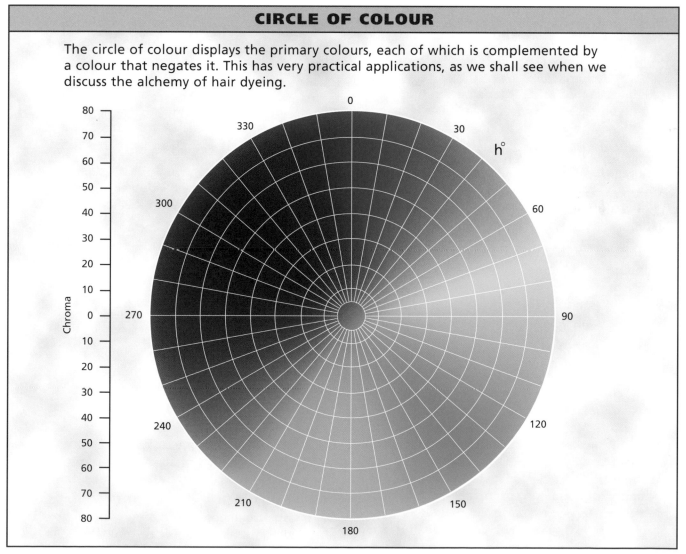

CIRCLE OF COLOUR

The circle of colour displays the primary colours, each of which is complemented by a colour that negates it. This has very practical applications, as we shall see when we discuss the alchemy of hair dyeing.

The colour circle.

Individual variation

The basics of colour vision are the same for everyone, but there are many variations between individuals. Moreover, after the age of 50 colour vision inevitably but slowly deteriorates.

SCIENCE BOX

Rods and cones

There are some 7 million cones and 120 million rods in the human retina, but they are not equally distributed throughout the retina. Rods, sensitive to low light, are found towards the periphery of the eye. This is why it is easier to see something in dim light if one looks at it sideways rather than straight on – for example, try looking straight at a faint star, and then sideways.

SCIENCE BOX

Colour blindness

People with a certain type of classical colour blindness cannot differentiate between red and green because they have an inherited abnormality in the photopigments of their cone cells. There are also other inherited problems, where sufferers experience a more subtle difficulty in differentiation of hues.

Colour terminology

The subject of colour is both simple and complex.

Attempting to 'name' colours can only ever be an approximation, as the spectrum of white light is continuous, and colours merge into each other. Descriptions such as 'sky-blue', 'blood-red' and 'jet-black' are common linguistic ways of communicating these colours. The reference point for yellow, however, may vary from 'canary' to 'corn'.

This simple, broad-brush approach does not fully express our own view of different colours, nor does it meet the need to construct a scientific 'model' or scale to allow accurate exchange of information. This was, for instance, vital in the production of this book. In the beauty industry, if people are to be persuaded to make the gamble on selecting a particular shade of hair colorant they also need to be able to reproduce it reliably again and again.

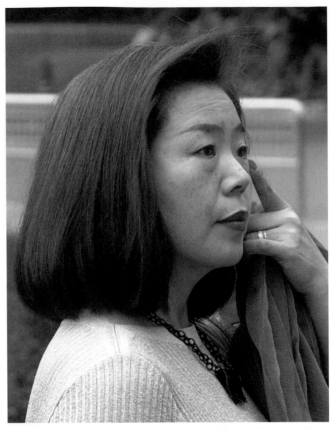

The buyer who carefully selects a shade of hair colorant relies on being able to reproduce its effect again and again. Science can measure this (see below).

Four basic terms are used in the description of the attributes of colour perception:

- **Brightness** describes the amount of light entering the eye. The eye is more sensitive to green than blue or red. This is why if different colours are viewed simultaneously under identical illumination, then for samples of equal colour saturation green appears the brightest.

- **Hue** describes a colour. All colours can be described by using combinations of red, blue, green and yellow (these four are called the **psychological primary colours**) in different ratios.

- **Saturation** is a measure of how much colour an object contains. The more saturated a colour, the more sensation is from light of a single wavelength.

- **Chroma** is the colourfulness of an object compared to white. It is very similar to saturation.

Colour systems

For the application of colour in the cosmetic industry, not only measurement of colour is significant but also the determination of colour differences.

It is important to customers that they obtain a reliable and reproducible hair colour product on each separate occasion of purchase. As we will see, colour charts for hair products incorporate all the above elements.

The CIE La*b* system is the result of work done in 1931 by the Commission Internationale d'Eclairage (CIE) and is the most commonly used so-called Colour Space System, based on human perception of colour using the three colour receptors. Within the CIE system every colour is assigned a 'formula'. It is assumed that three sets of signals are triggered to the brain:

- light or dark
- red or green
- yellow or blue.

They are opposing in that a given receptor receives, say, a red signal or a green one but not both. This Opponent Ypte Colour space number is derived mathematically from the CIE values in the following manner.

L = measure of lightness of an object – values range from 0 (black) to 100 (white)
A = measure of redness (positive a) or greenness (negative a)
B = measure of yellowness (positive b) or blueness (negative b)

A more recent development is the CIELCH or more simply LCH system. It employs the same system as the CIE La*b* colour space but describes the location of colour in space by use of polar coordinates rather than rectangular coordinates, where:

L = measure of lightness and has a value between 0 and 100
C = measure of chroma (saturation) and represents the distance from the neutral axis
H = measure of hue and is represented as an angle ranging from 0 to 360°.

Angles 0–90° are reds, oranges and yellows.
90–180° are yellows, yellow-greens and greens
180–270° are greens, blue-greens and blues
270–360° are blues, purples and magentas and return to red.

These complicated systems are important in the industrial production of hair dyes.

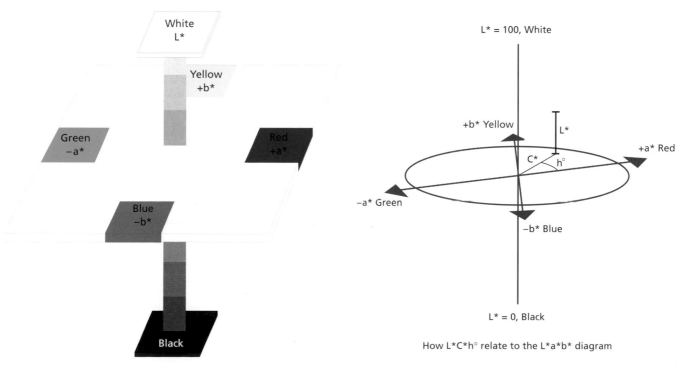

*The CIE system La *b* of denoting colours.*

The CIE LCH system.

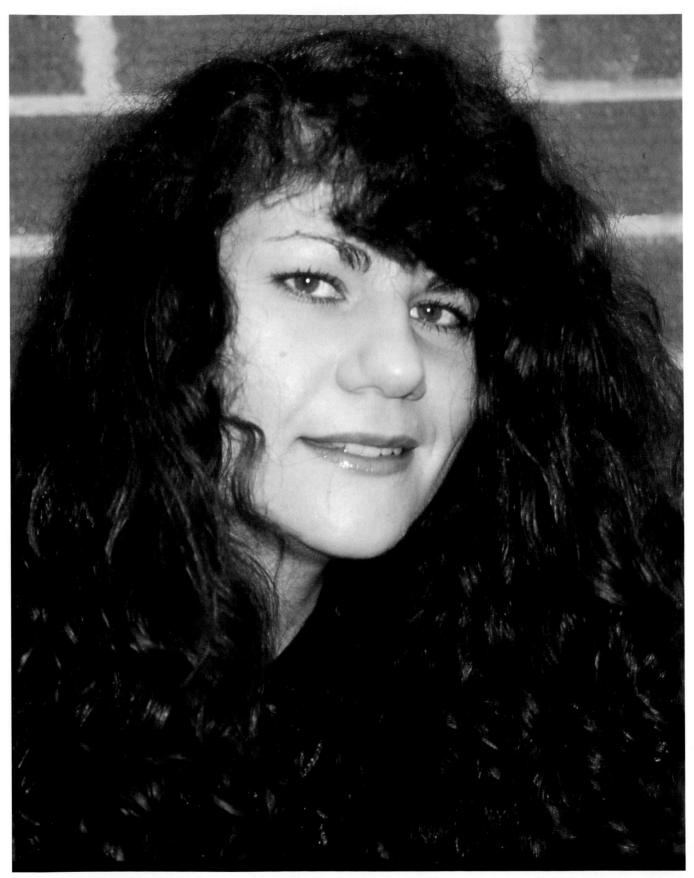

'Raven tresses' loaded with melanin.

3

Hair pigments and the hair follicle

The hair follicle is an extraordinarily complex organ, and is capable of manufacturing almost every known hormone and natural chemical messengers (mediators) found in the rest of the body. The follicle is influenced by many internal factors (and possible external and environmental factors too) that impact on its otherwise steady production of pigmented hair.

It is now apparent that the hair follicle does not produce just one pigment at the same concentration throughout our lives. In childhood pigment concentration in the hair is low and increases particularly after puberty. In addition not *all* follicles in an individual necessarily produce the same pigment. Some may produce eumelanin, others phaeomelanin (see below). This may in some cases account for brunettes.

Human hairs do not grow synchronously, and each follicle or group of follicles may bear a hair(s) of different 'quality' and pigmentary status from its neighbours.

Hair colour pigments

Hair colour is due to the presence of unique natural chemicals – melanins – in the cortex of the hair. The production of these pigments is inherited under the influence of at least four gene positions (loci), which are probably allelic.

Most human hair is black or dark brown in colour. Groups of genes express (control the production of) a special dark pigment called **eumelanin**. This pigment is genetically dominant, that is, it is expressed in preference to pigments of lighter shades in each follicle.

Light and red shades are due to the presence of a specific melanin known as **phaeomelanin**, which is a 'mutation' of eumelanin.

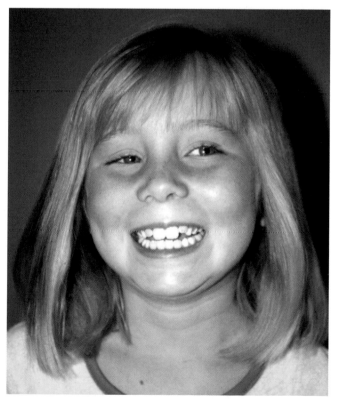

Light shades of hair, due to the presence of phaeomelanin.

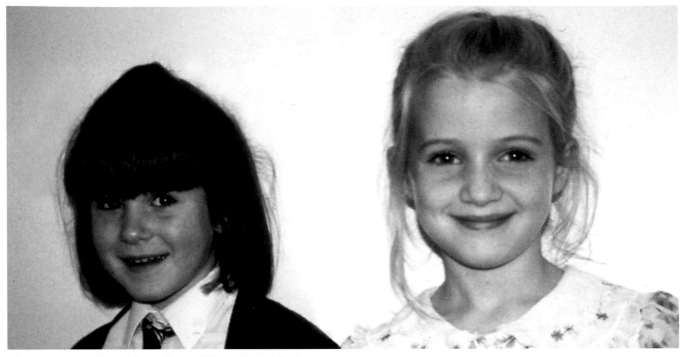

These two sisters have inherited very different genes for hair colour.

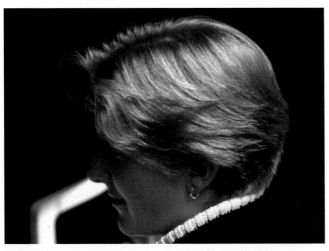

We do not yet know the genetic coding for blonde hair.

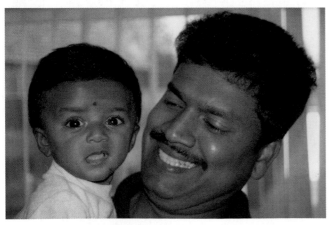

Dark and dominant black hair.

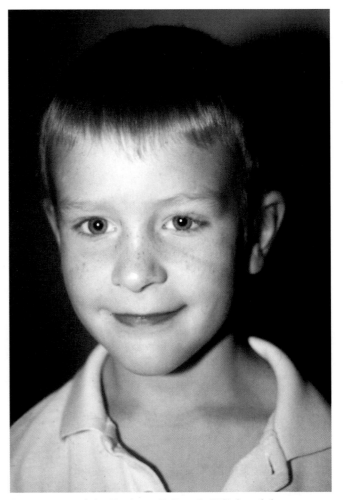

Recent research by Professor J. Rees in Edinburgh has elucidated the inheritance mechanism of red hair.

Hair colour from the follicle to the tip

The natural pigments of hair are formed in specialized cells, the **melanocytes**, deep within the hair follicle. These are found in the germinative part of the hair – the hair bulb.

The melanocyte

Melanocytes are specialized pigment-producing cells in the dermal papilla of the hair bulb. They are hidden among the germinative cells of the hair matrix and are in close contact with the basement membrane.

Melanocytes are also present in the external root sheath and are derived from the areas in the developing foetus responsible for the nervous system, the neural crest.

Pigment in the hair bulb

Melanocytes secrete tiny packages of pigments called **melanosomes**. The process involves a complex of proteins and depends on the enzyme tyrosinase and other auxiliary enzymes.

The melanosomes are distributed within the cytoplasm of the melanocytes, close to the nucleus of the cell. Melanocytes possess slender extensions (**dendrites**) which deliver these pigment packages into the cells of the germinative epithelium in the hair bulb.

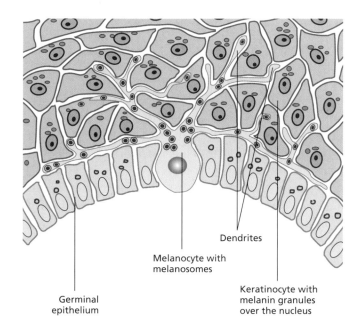

The development of melanin in melanocytes. Not every keratinocyte receives pigment.

[*Source* Thomson Learning – World of Skin Care]

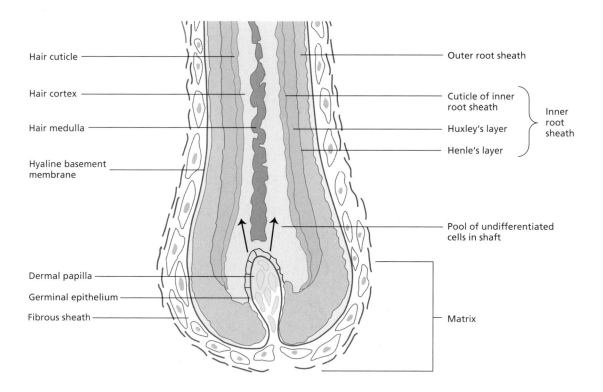

The structure of the hair bulb: the living cells gradually die and are compressed to form the hair shaft.

[*Source* Thomson Learning – World of Skin Care]

Pigment is destined for the cells of the cortex: no pigment is deposited in the cells that will form the cuticle and the internal root sheath cells – although pigment granules have been detected in the cuticle of human nostril hair!

In black hair, the deposition of melanin (within melanosomes) in the hair bulb continues until the whole unit is uniformly dense. Lighter coloured hair shows less melanin deposition and blonde shows melanosomes that are much less uniform. The melanosomes of red and blonde hair are spherical: in black and brown hair they are ellipsoidal.

It is not certain whether melanocytes choose only certain cells in which to deposit pigment, and if so, how the selection is made. Sections in some hairs may show lines of pigment in apparent strict regimentation, but other hairs on the same head do not necessarily carry this pattern.

Towards the end of the active growing phase (**anagen**), while the growing hair cells (keratinoctytes) are still proliferating, the melanocytes retract their dendrites and cease producing melanosomes. This heralds the movement into the transitional phase of hair growth (**catagen**) and marks a reduction in the activity of the enzyme tyrosinase. This can be seen in the pigment-free bulb of the shed hair.

During the resting phase of the hair cycle (**telogen**) the melanocytes remain at the surface of the papilla in a shrunken form.

The genetic regulation of the process of hair pigmentation is probably exerted at several points along the 'pigmentory pathway'. This includes influencing how the behaviour of the basic pigment cells – the migration of the melanocytes to the hair bulb, their subsequent proliferation and the interactions between the melanocyte and the dermis in the hair bulb.

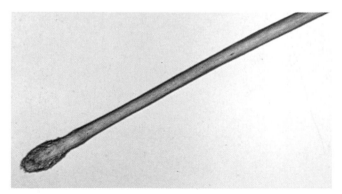

Pigment-free bulb of a shed hair.

[*Source* Thomson Learning – The World of Hair]

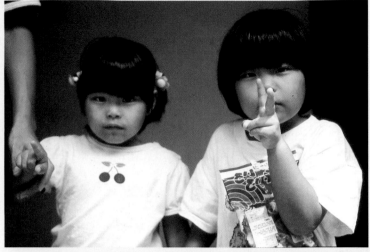

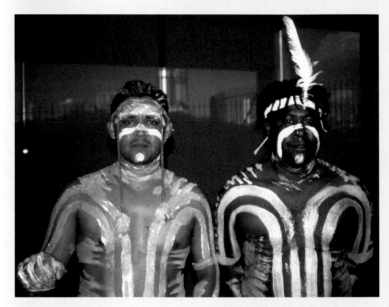

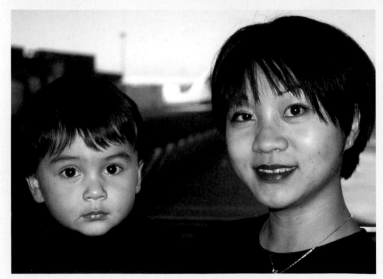

Mother's dark hair determines her Anglo-Chinese child's colour.

CHINA

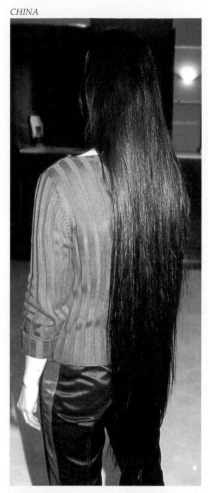

CAPE TOWN

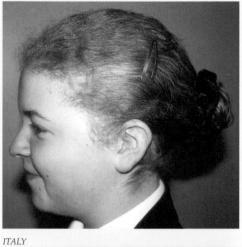

ITALY

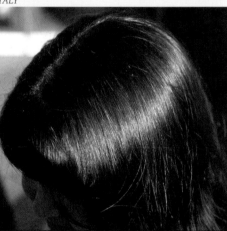

LATIN AMERICA

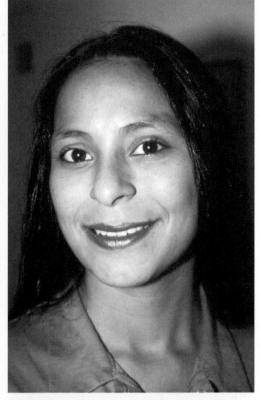

SCANDINAVIA

AFRICA

IRAN

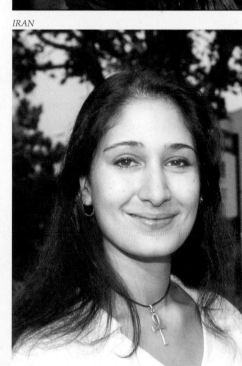

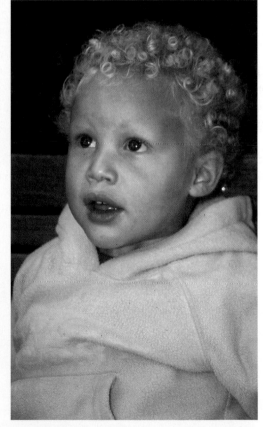

The growth and pigmentation seen in human hair can be affected by various factors, including racial and sex differences, variable response to hormones and age-related changes.

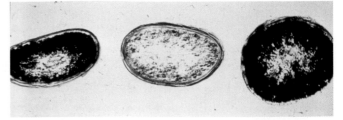

African, European and Oriental hair showing pigment deposition: the different pigments and distribution around the periphery of the cortex can be seen.

Pigment in the hair shaft

In the hair shaft melanin granules are distributed throughout the cortex, which forms the bulk of the hair shaft, but show the greatest concentration towards the edge (periphery).

Structure of melanin

Melanins are the result of a series of reactions in which there is progressive oxidation of the amino-acid tyrosine. They exist as granules that are generally in the range of 0.2–0.8 μ in length and constitute less than 3% of hair mass.

Natural melanins usually exist bound to protein and cannot be made soluble without degradation. They tend to bind to other colours very easily and probably do not form crystalline structures.

Traditionally melanin has been regarded as a high-molecular-weight amorphous polymer (a very large molecule) of linked carboxylic acid units.

A more recent suggestion is that melanin consists of an aggregation of tiny fundamental particles called 'proto-molecules' of dimension 15Å. These fundamental particles are comprised of 5DHI/DHICA oligomer (small polymer) units that self-assemble in three or four layers.

These fundamental particles subsequently aggregate in the pigment granule. This process is influenced by the presence of metal ions, especially copper, and the protein backbone in the melanin granule.

Melanocytes produce melanins in response to the melanocyte-stimulating hormone (MSH), which is produced in the pituitary gland, the effect of which is to darken lightly coloured hair. MSH acts on a special receptor, the **melanocortin 1 receptor** or MC1R (Rees 2000).

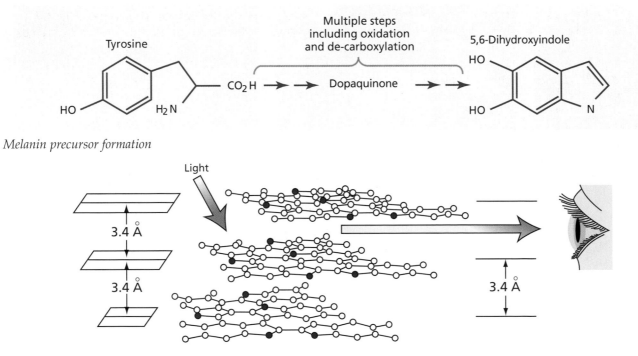

Melanin precursor formation

Melanin probably consists of an aggregation of 'proto-molecules'; light passing through these molecules is partially absorbed and refracted to produce the 'colour' we see.

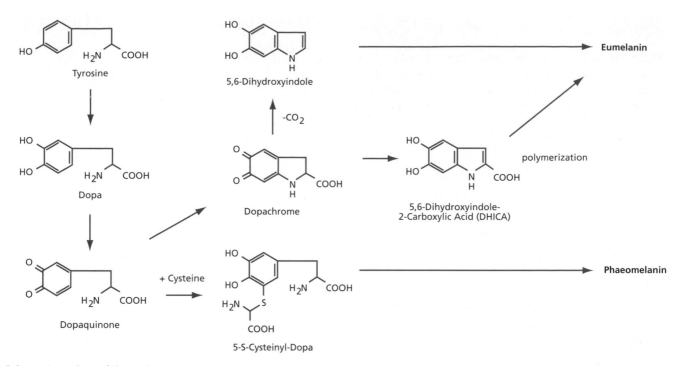

Schematic outline of the melanogenic pathway, showing the major intermediates of both eumelanin and phaeomelanin.

SCIENCE BOX

Eumelanin

Eumelanin is a polymer of irregular structure, often conjugated to proteins, which is derived from tyrosine, dopa and possibly dopamine.

In the presence of the enzyme tyrosinase and molecular oxygen, melanin is produced via intermediate substances that play an important role in the regulation of the melanin synthesis pathway in the hair bulb. In the case of eumelanin, decarboxylation of dopachrome gives the intermediate 5,6-dihydroxyindole, which together with dihydroxyindolecarboxylic acid (DHIAC) is the immediate precursor of melanin. Oxidative polymerization of DHIAC probably completes the process.

Eumelanins are insoluble in most solvents and resist chemical treatment.

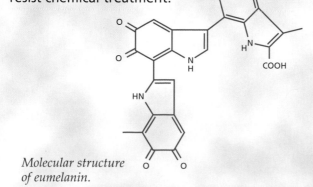

Molecular structure of eumelanin.

SCIENCE BOX

Phaeomelanins

The group of pigments known as phaeomelanins includes polymers containing benzothiazole and tetrahydroisoquinolone together with minor pigments based on 2',2'-bis(1,4-benzothiazine).

These pigments occur in nature by modification of the eumelanin pathway, which involves an interaction of dopaquinone with cysteine. It is probable that the melanocortin 1 receptor is key to the control in melanogenesis. Loss of function by mutations of MC1R are associated with a switch from eumelanin to phaeomelanin resulting in red or yellow pigmentation.

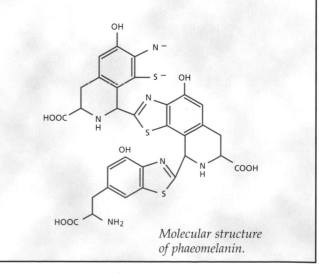

Molecular structure of phaeomelanin.

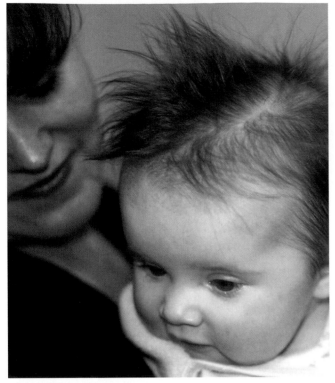

New born babies often have dark, soft, fine hair, bearing little resemblance to that of their parents. This is embryonic (lanugo) hair representing millions of years of evolution.

Pigmentation from youth to old age

Some individuals may be capable of producing both hair pigments and in differing concentrations at various times in their lives, which may explain why a dramatic colour change is often seen over the years from birth to old age. Hair seen at birth – the so-called **lanugo** hair – is frequently dark and prolific. It is shed sooner or later after birth to be replaced by hair that is often of a different hue and form.

The early childhood hair of native Australian Aborigines, for example, may be unexpectedly light, only darkening after puberty. Childhood phaeomelanin-pigmented hair is often white-blonde, only to darken to a mid-brown by adulthood.

The much more prevalent eumelanin hair can be a lighter brown in youth, only to darken with the onset of puberty.

The gradual emergence of unpigmented hair with advancing years is very common, until in extreme old age white is almost universal. We discuss the significance of grey hair later in this chapter.

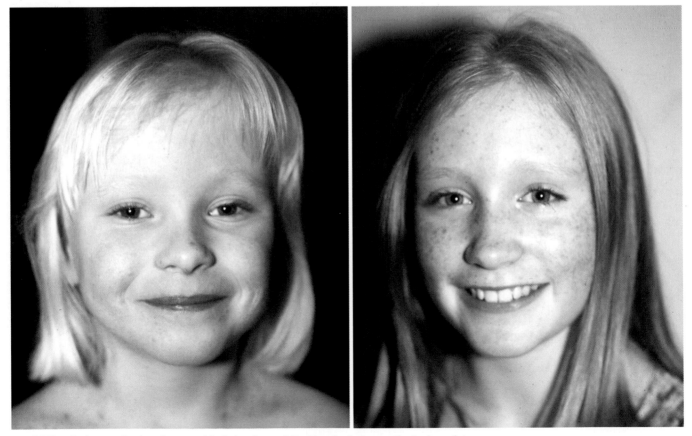

In childhood phaeomelanin-pigmented hair is often white-blonde, but usually darkens later.

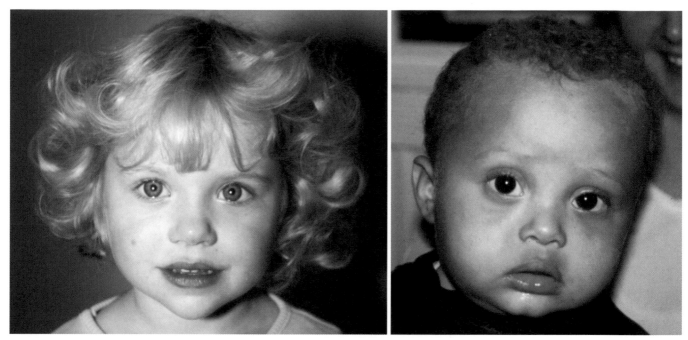

Hair in childhood frequently shows not only lighter shades but often different hair form (curls) too.

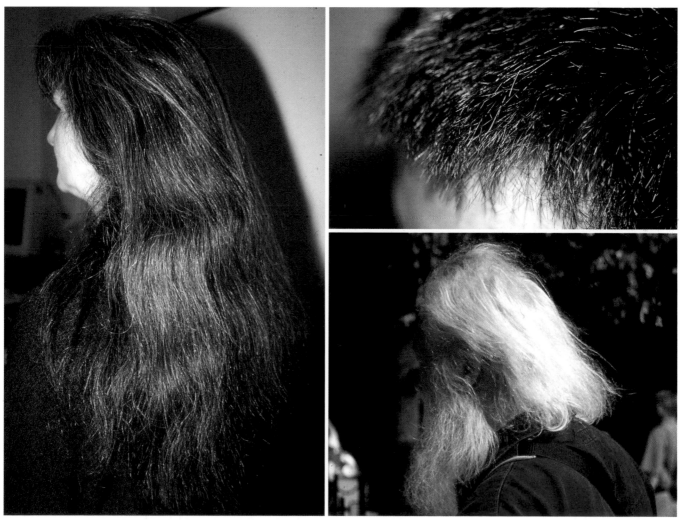

In older people the gradual loss of pigmented hair is epidemic.

Hair colour

Hair colour and light reflection

The colours of all natural pigments lie in a narrow segment of the Commission Internationale d'Eclairage Colour Space corresponding to reflection of the wavelengths between 586 and 606 nm.

Reflectance varies over a wide range, from 2% for black hair to 90% for albino hair. Here are some reflectance facts:

- 'Virgin' brown hair (i.e. hair that has never been treated by chemicals or heat) shows a featureless absorption in the visible region that steadily increases in the red region. This curve changes as a function of hair colour (dark brown, mid-brown, light brown) as seen below. Hair with no melanin (natural white hair) has a different profile.

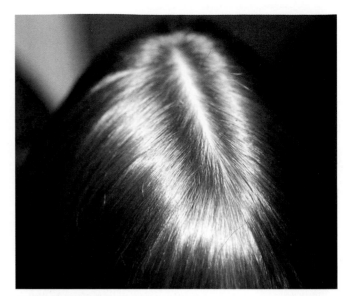

'Virgin' brown hair showing reflectance.

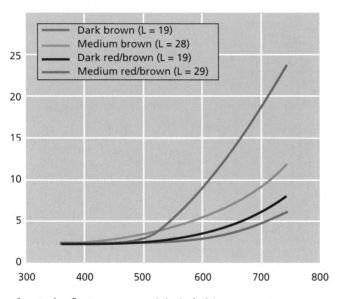

Spectral reflectance curves (virgin hair). [Source P & G data on file]

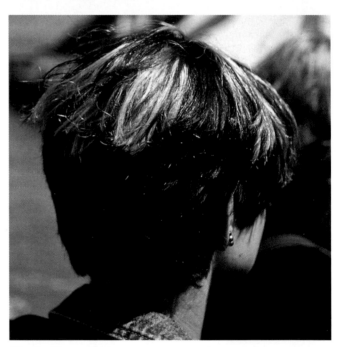

Bleached brown hair.

- Virgin red hair: The spectral reflectance curves for red hair as compared with brown hair show a clear increase in the reflectance at the red end of the spectrum.

- Bleached brown hair: On bleaching the spectral reflectance curves show an increase in reflectance in the red region.

- For lighter hair the shape of the curves change slightly on bleaching, and are then possibly dominated more by absorption due to keratin than to melanin.

- Bleached red hair: The bleaching profile of red hair (with say, ammonium hydroxide/ hydrogen peroxide) is very different from that of brown hair and may hold the key to the melanin bleaching process. Instead of a large difference in lightness (L) on the first cycle of bleaching, there is little difference in L on the first but a large difference between cycles 1 and 3.

Phaeomelanin may be more resistant to bleaching than eumelanin is, but this question is as yet unresolved.

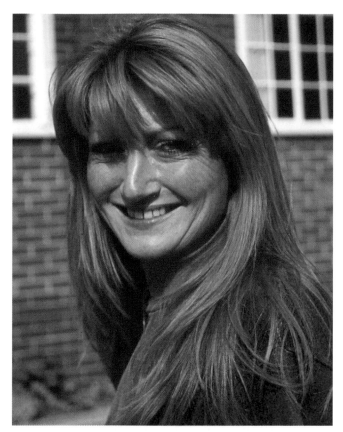

Bleached red hair.

Loss of hair pigments

Pigments deposited in the maturing hair shaft are naturally carried upwards to emerge into the 'full light of day'. Their effect is immediately seen.

Over time, however, the effects of ultra-violet radiation result in degradation of the amino-acids that make up the melanosomes and a consequent subtle loss of colour. This is most commonly seen in long hair and is accentuated by chemical treatment.

The root-to-tip difference can be quite marked and is associated with natural and accelerated ageing.

Weathering

Colour may be gradually lost from the hair shaft during everyday 'living'. This is part of the so-called **weathering** process wherein the structure and normal physiological functions of the hair deteriorate. This has implications for the pigmentation of the hair.

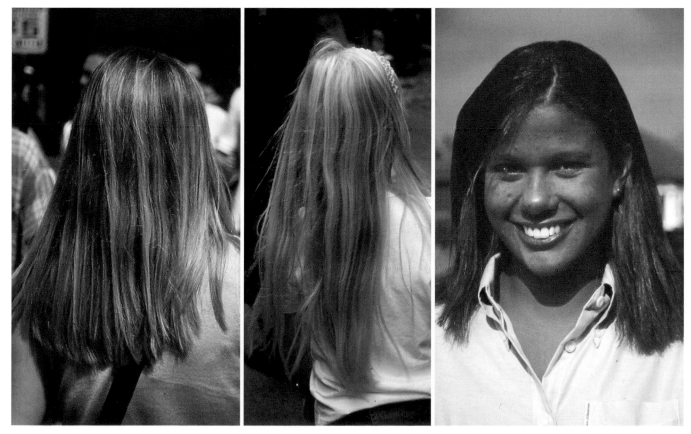

The root-to-tip difference in pigmentation and reflectance can be marked.

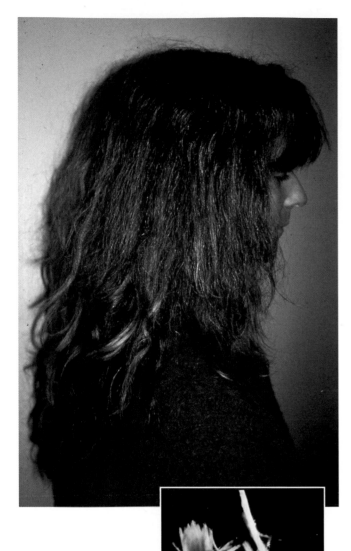

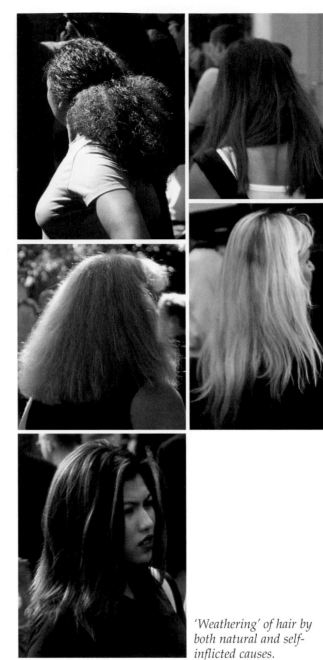

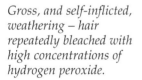

Gross, and self-inflicted, weathering – hair repeatedly bleached with high concentrations of hydrogen peroxide.

'Weathering' of hair by both natural and self-inflicted causes.

We have all observed the effects of sunlight on hair after prolonged sun exposure. Hair 'weathers' along its length, and over time the cortex and the cuticle may become disrupted.

These defects of the hair shaft may affect the appearance of the colour as seen through the hair shaft, particularly at the tips where maximal weathering occurs. Dark hair is lightened to brownish-red and (rarely) to blonde even after prolonged high exposure to the ultra-violet. Brown hair may be bleached white, but there may be serious consequences for its quality.

Grey hair

Grey hair may merely reflect a genetically regulated exhaustion of the melanocyte reservoir's potential, or perhaps some defect in cells activating migration. Some hair scientists support a hypothesis of greying hair that suggests that free-radical damage to the DNA of the germinal epithelium leads to mutations.

The loss of hair pigmentation – greying or **canities**, in technical terms – affects us all in time to a greater or lesser degree. The onset and

NEW YORK

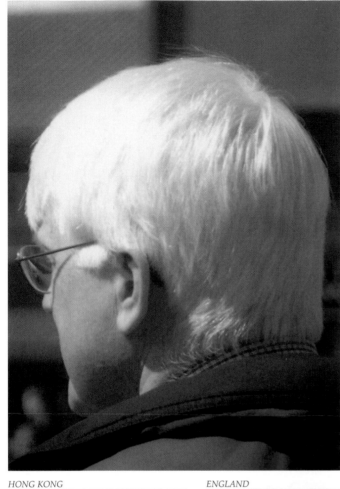

DENMARK

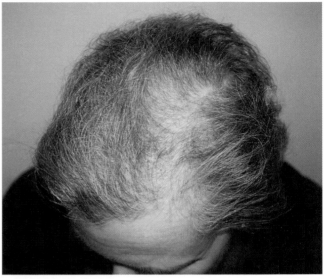

WASHINGTON

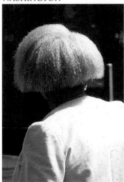

CAPE TOWN

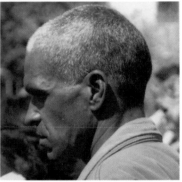

HONG KONG

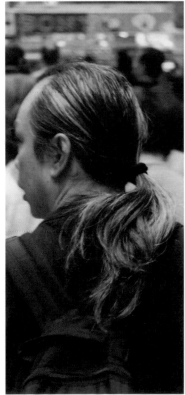

ENGLAND

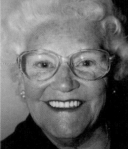

ENGLAND

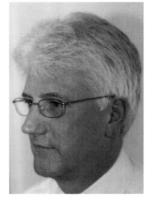

AUSTRALIA

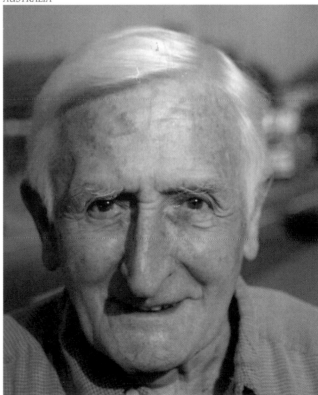

Greying around the world.

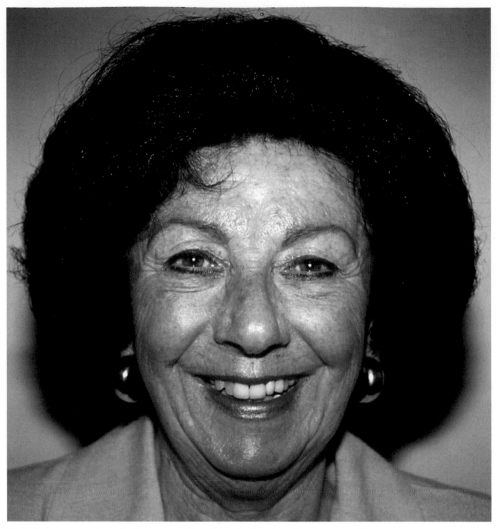

This lady cannot bear to be seen without her hair colouring to cover the grey.

progression of hair greying is closely associated with so-called 'chronological' ageing and occurs to varying degrees in all individuals, regardless of sex or ethnic group. No head is immune, even if only the occasional or solitary hair changes colour.

Grey hair does, however, appear to be inherited as an autosomal dominant character. The age of onset of greying also appears to be inherited: entire families may show significant early greying. The average age for Indo-Europeans is the mid-thirties, for Orientals the late thirties and for Africans the mid-forties. Hair is said to grey prematurely if grey hair appears before the age of 20 in Indo-Europeans, before 25 in Asians and before 30 in Africans. The progress of greying is entirely individual, although by 50 years of age, 50% of European people have 50% grey hair.

This greying results not from the failure or extermination of all the hair follicle melanocytes, but specifically of those located in the melanogenic zone of the hair follicle. Some melanocytes without pigment (said to be **amelanotic**) are retained in the outer root sheath and sebaceous gland of follicles bearing white hairs. While the functions of outer root sheath amelanotic melanocytes in hair and skin biology are as yet far from clear, they are available for repigmentation and repopulation of the epidermis if necessary (after skin wounding, for example).

Their lack of contribution in hair pigmentation may indicate that this location in the so-called 'senile' white hair follicle does not allow for migration to the melanogenic zone during early hair growth (anagen), as apparently occurs in pigment-producing follicles. Hair

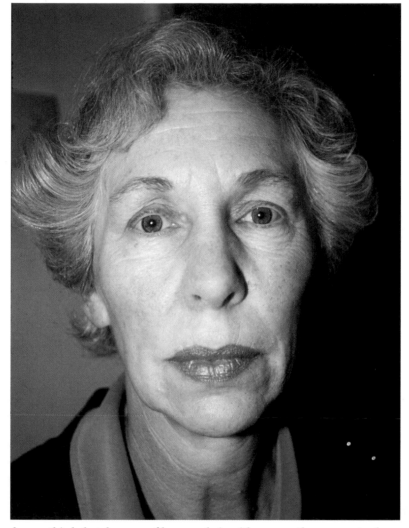

…whereas this lady takes care of her grey hair with apparently no urge to change it.

repigmentation can be induced by, for instance, radiation therapy for cancer or after inflammatory events such as wounds. It is probable that this results from radiation/cytokine-induced activation of melanocytes in the hair follicle reservoir, and may suggest that melanocytes might be induced to migrate and develop (differentiate) to repigment greying hair follicles naturally.

What, however, is the extent of greying and what is the evolutionary significance? Why in so many cultures is there such desire to cover it?

SCIENCE BOX

At age 50, 50% of all people are likely to have 50% grey hair.

Grey hairs are always more apparent among dark hairs, and the distribution is different in dark-haired and blonde peoples.

Skin changes due to ageing in humans are associated with a 10–20% reduction in pigment-producing melanocytes, whether in exposed or unexposed skin, for every decade after 30 years of age. There is a body-wide loss of tyrosinase-positive melanocytes, not only from the epidermis but also from the hair follicle, moles (naevi) and the eye. While this decrease results in gradual loss of colour from the skin, age-related loss in the colour of hair is much more dramatic, suggesting a different 'melanocyte clock' in the hair pigmentary unit.

It has been suggested that cigarette smoking may be linked with premature greying and even hair loss, raising the spectre of greying as a marker for general health status. A possible

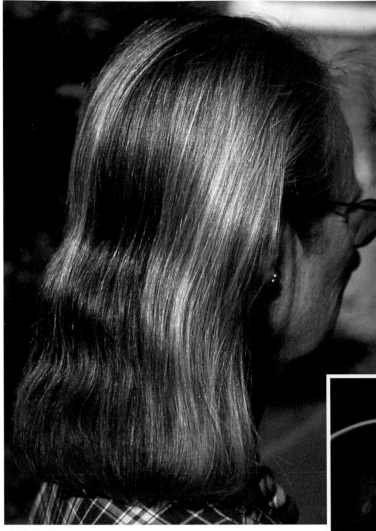

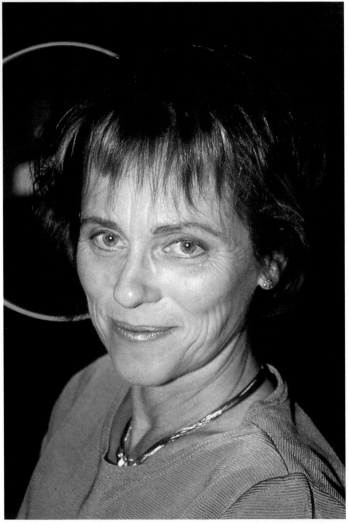

*A spectacular transformation –
covering the grey. A fantastic cut
and creation from a top stylist
and products.*

SCIENCE BOX

The nature of grey hair

Grey hair is coarser, wirier and less manageable than pigmented hair, it is often unable to hold a permanent or temporary set and is more resistant to artificial colour. Both of these observations suggest significant change to the underlying substructure of the hair shaft. In this way, ageing hair follicles may reprogram their matrix cells to increase production of medullary, rather than cortical, keratinocytes (the medulla is often enlarged and collapsed, forming a central cavity in grey and white hairs).

explanation of the above may be that smoking-related diseases accelerate the ageing of many body systems, including pigmentation.

In species such as cattle copper deficiency causes **achromotrichia** (the production of unpigmented hair), since copper is an essential part of the tyrosinase molecule. In humans, however, abnormal hair coloration due to dietary deficiencies is rare, though not unknown.

Hair colour changes are a prominent feature in conditions of protein malnutrition, such as kwashiorkor. Normal black hair becomes brown or reddish, and brown hair becomes blonde. Intermittent protein malnutrition leads to the 'flag' sign of kwashiorkor: alternating white (abnormal) and dark bands occur along individual hairs.

The lightening of hair colour from black to brown observed in severe iron-deficiency anaemia may be an effect on keratinization rather than on melanocyte function. Browning of dark hair may also be seen in kidney disease (nephrotic syndrome).

Accidental hair discoloration

Hair avidly binds inorganic elements, and hair colour changes are occasionally seen after exposure to certain substances.

Exposure of blonde hair to high concentrations of copper in tap water (usually from new pipes) or swimming pools may result in green hair. This is only visible in hair that has been heavily processed.

Cobalt workers may develop bright blue hair, whilst a deep blue tint has been seen in indigo handlers. A yellow hair colour is not uncommon in white- or grey-haired heavy smokers; it is due to the tar in cigarette smoke. Yellow staining may also occur from picric acid and dithranol.

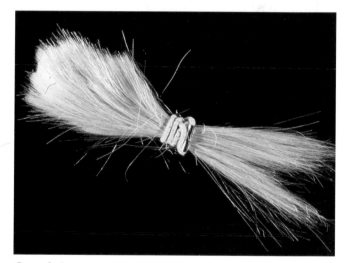

Green hair.

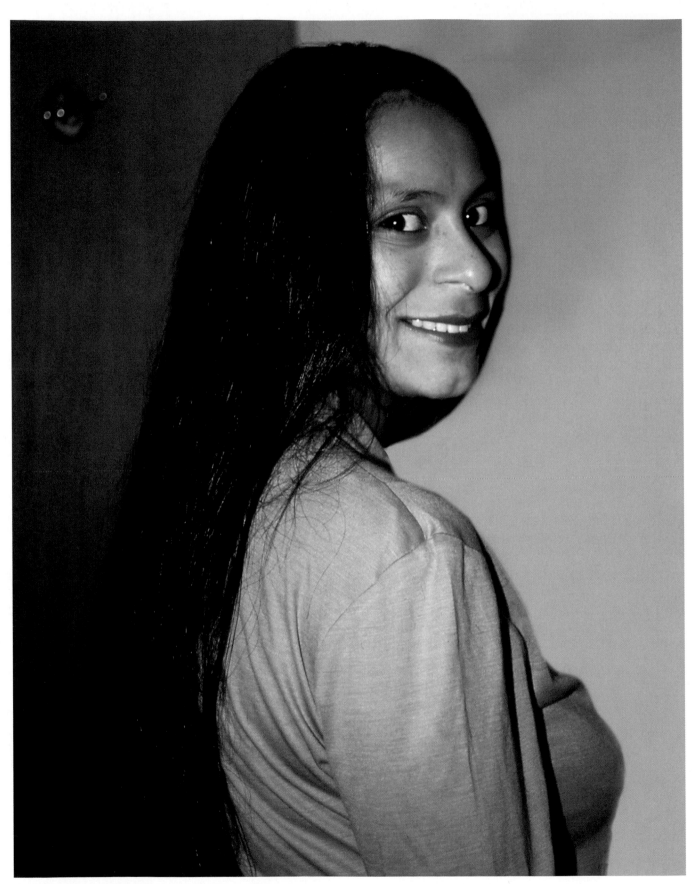

A native of Peru: black hair, in superlative condition.

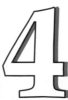

Human hair colour in history

Although black and dark brown hair dominate the world, the range of skin and eye colours varies since hair, skin and eye colour are due to the expression of different groups of genes. The widely separated peoples of Kashmir and Ireland have a frequent expression of dark hair and blue eyes, denoting their joint origins as Indo-European peoples who migrated north and west in late Neolithic times.

The large and relatively static population of Greater China has a more uniform colour expression. Korean and Japanese people (apart from the Ainu, who inhabit the northernmost island) are genetically closely similar and display much the same characteristics.

Most of the populations of southern Asia are descendants of Asiatic peoples migrating from the southern rim of China and eventually reaching the Polynesian islands. Native Americans are descended from Asian peoples who intermittently reached North America via Alaska. Eventually humankind reached the tip of South America around 12 000 years ago. All these peoples are dark-haired.

Offshoots of the Indo-European peoples reaching north-west Europe as recently as 35 000 years ago probably carried a mutated eumelanin gene responsible for phaeomelanin production in sufficient quantity to allow the developing and static farming communities which eventually emerged after the last ice age to express it in significant numbers.

Moving closer to our own times, the waves of migration to North and South America after 1492 took all hair types and colour to the New World.

In North America only some 5% of people have naturally blonde hair – much the same proportion as in western Europe.

Hair colour and its social implications

Although relatively short, the recorded history of humanity does give an abiding impression of the manner in which hair colour has been viewed and used in the social interactions of the day.

The Greeks thought that red hair was a sign of bad luck and even of barbarism, which may have reflected their view of the warlike Celtic tribes of central Europe. These peoples were eventually either incorporated into the Roman Empire or forced into its western fringes. (In later centuries when the Scots made up the core

MALAYSIA

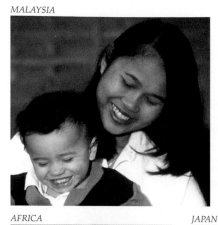

LONDON

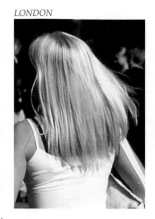

CHINA

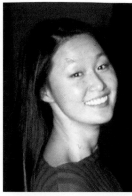

MOROCCO

AFRICA

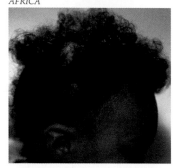

JAPAN

PORTUGAL

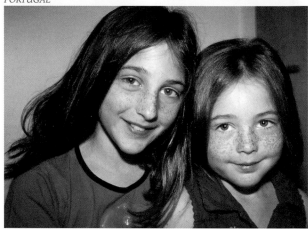

DENMARK

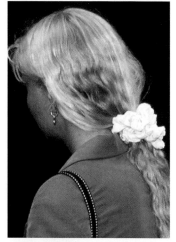

ITALY

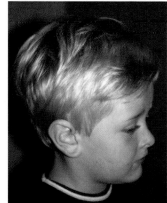

GERMANY

CHINA

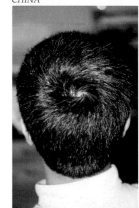

ROMANY

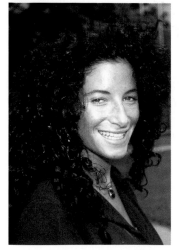

ANGLO-CARRIBBEAN

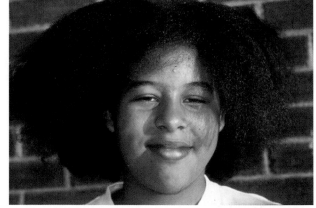

95% of all humans have dark hair – blondes are relatively 'rare' exceptions.

Hair as signal

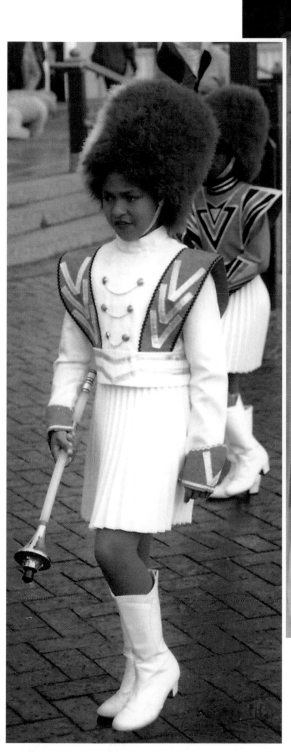

The green busby represents hair which sends
a strong signal to others in her group.

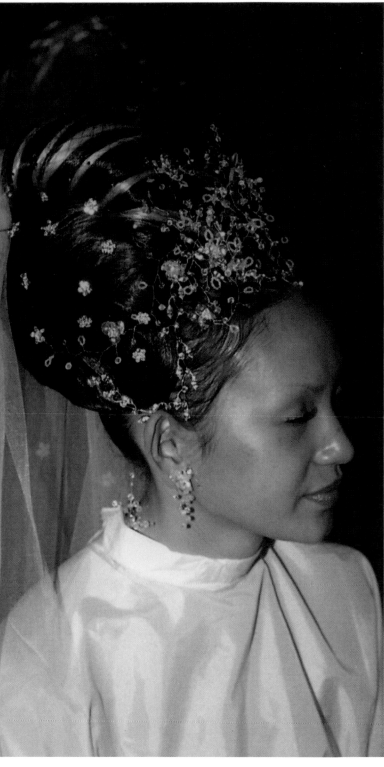

*Elaborate style and colour on that most
glorious of days sends a strong signal of
'bride'.*

of the British Imperial army, their bravery and ferocity became synonymous with red hair.)

In the early Christian world, children with golden hair were regarded with reverence, particularly in regions where this colouring was rare. It is said that an early Pontiff seeing captive northern children exclaimed *'non Angli sunt sed angeli'*, translated as 'they are not Angles but angels', thus adding to the mystic significance which perhaps reflected the older animistic religions.

From the Middle Ages onwards artists customarily portrayed the traitor Judas with red hair. In England, admiration of the hair of Queen Elizabeth I changed the national attitude to red hair, however.

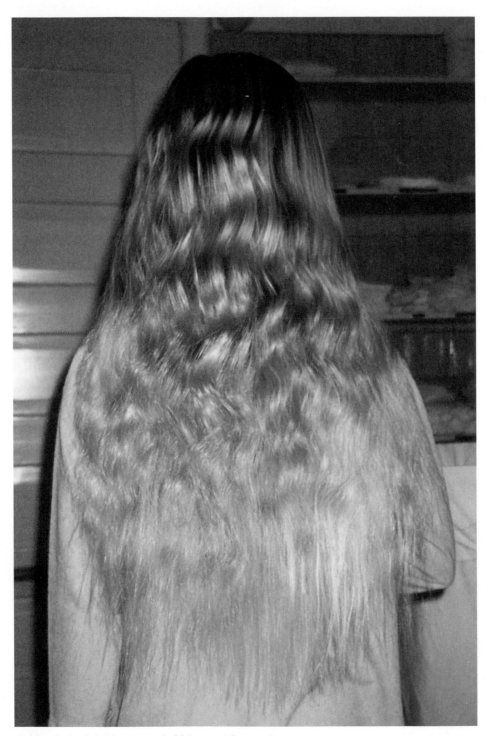

Golden-haired children were held in special regard.

Botticelli's Venus assisted the further international rehabilitation of this unique colour. The pre-Raphaelites frequently showed their idealized young women with long red or auburn hair, and in late Victorian times it became highly fashionable.

In the 20th century the explosion of the communications media, particularly the cinema and more recently television, had a powerful global influence on style and fashion, and particularly on hair styles and 'in' colours. In the less politically correct Hollywood of the twenties, thirties and forties stereotypical images of hair abounded. 'Blondes have most fun,' it was said, 'redheads are fiery and brunettes are cool and sophisticated.'

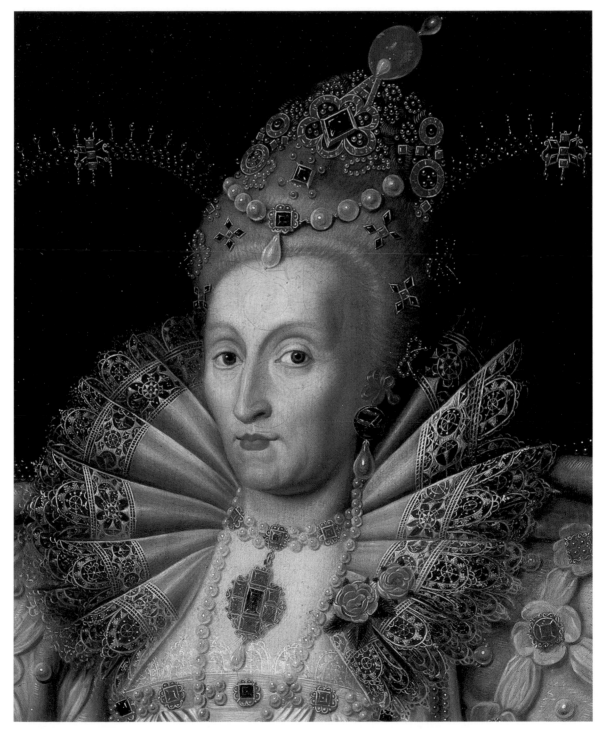

Admiration of the hair of Queen Elizabeth I changed the English national attitude to red hair.

[*Source* Thomson Learning – The World of Skin Care]

LONDON

NEW YORK

HONG KONG

LONDON

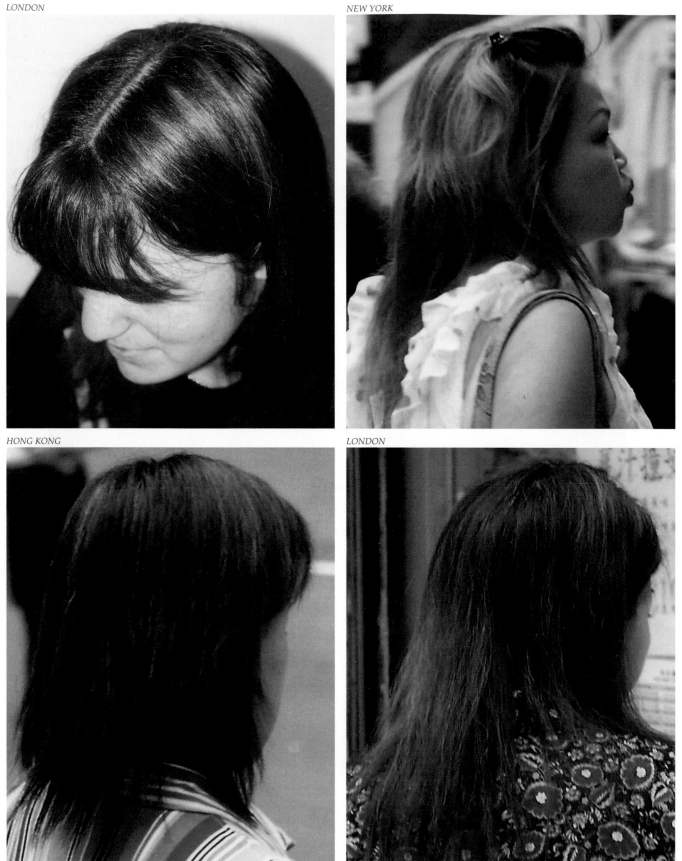

In black hair, in order to effect a colour change, the dense pigment is oxidized. This results in the appearance of the next colour in sequence – red.

Black, brunette, red and blonde

In her famous book *The Vogue Book of Blondes*, the doyenne of fashion Kathy Phillips described the current obsession with blonde – *the* hair colour of the 20th century – fuelled by female (and to a lesser extent male) movie stars. Here we look at the significance of the different human hair colours in the past and in today's world.

Black

Black-haired icons of the last 100 years such as Muhammed Ali, Audrey Hepburn, Che Guevara, Sean Connery, Tom Cruise, Nelson Mandela and Whoopi Goldberg, each an enormously significant impact on global perception.

Black and dark-brown hues are expressed in every continent by the presence of the pigment eumelanin, although in differing concentrations. Shades vary from a deep almost matt black to blue-black to dark brown.

The genetic inheritance is well understood and its expression is dominant.

Does black hair have any particular evolutionary or social significance? We are but the fifth member of an exclusive line of mammals – the great apes, among whom darkly pigmented hair predominates. In our ancestral homeland of Africa and during the expansion into the Arabian peninsula and onward into Asia and Australasia, the dark pigment would have continued to protect people from the sun. Over succeeding generations this pigment was carried into the four corners of the earth (see the map on page 9). It is no surprise that over 90% of the world's inhabitants have dark hair.

In women smooth, shining dark hair, as exemplified by Audrey Hepburn – recently voted the most beautiful woman (ever) in the world – epitomizes elegance and beauty. In the Western world it is often associated with 'passion' and spirit, while in the East it is synonymous with delicate beauty.

The possession of black hair may be a cause of envy to those with more indeterminate hues, but many women with black hair, finding themselves at one extreme of the pigment spectrum, wish to move to the other. In this market place, the impact of Hollywood stars should not be underestimated.

In order to effect a colour change in black hair, the dense pigment must be removed, and that can be achieved only by oxidizing it. A colour shift naturally results in the next colour in sequence – red. This result is widely seen in the Orient, where the younger generation follows fashion and pop idols. As a result of repeated bleaching hair quality can suffer, with hair becoming dry and lustreless.

Red hair

On a global basis naturally red hair is much less common than other shades, but is the most popular 'fun' shade.

As we have seen, the melanin pigment responsible for the colour in red hair is phaeomelanin. It is strongly linked to blood group O. Genetic studies in the UK and Italy have shown that the distribution of red hair mirrors the presence of this group and the incidence of red hair varies from 0.3% in Germany to 3.7% in England and 11% in parts of Scotland.

In Africa reddish coloration can sometimes be seen, but not widely; it is generally assumed that this is evidence of the early mutation of tyrosine metabolism carried forward to subsequent generations. The issue is confused, however, by the potential for much later reintroduction of European genes during Colonial days. Only large studies of gene sequencing in the myriad ethnic groups in Africa could clarify this dichotomy.

THE DARK-HAIRED AND DESIRABLE HERO

In a social and mating context the archetypal male is classically cast as 'tall, dark and handsome'. A naturally sandy-haired Elvis dyed his hair black, and the rest is history.

Matt Ridley in his famous book *The Red Queen* argues that 'tall, dark and handsome' men are preferentially selected by women as representing strength and protection. Most authorities agree that, in contrast, a man tends to choose a mate who is lighter-skinned and (often in consequence) lighter-haired.

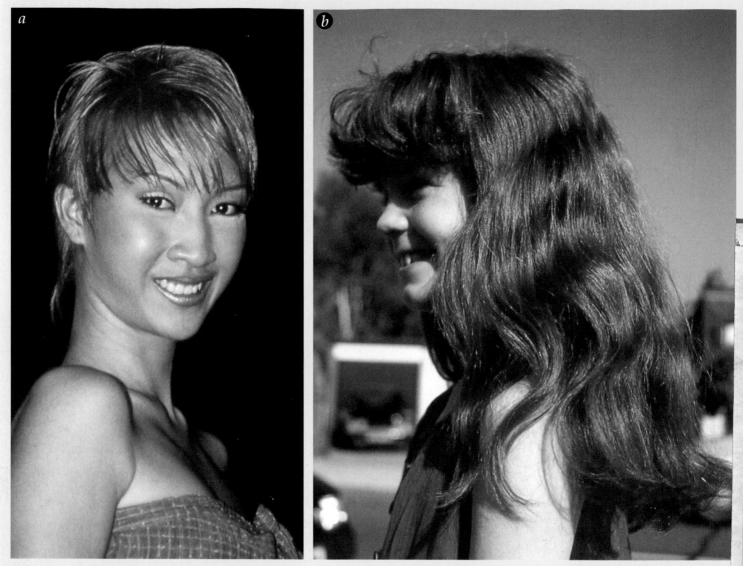

Red hair – art mimicking nature

SCIENCE BOX

Red hair inheritance follows a so-called homozygous recessive mechanism. That is, it requires the inheritance of the gene for red hair from both parents. Having only one red-haired parent is insufficient.

Based on DNA sequencing, the key control point in the production of red hair has been shown to be the melanocortin 1 receptor (MC1R) found on melanocytes and other cell types. Signalling via this receptor increases the proportion of eumelanin to phaeomelanin. Decreased signalling through this pathway results in red hair. The gene is associated with increased skin cancer risk, freckling and sun sensitivity.

The intensity of red hair coloration may vary over time, and the hair may darken with age.

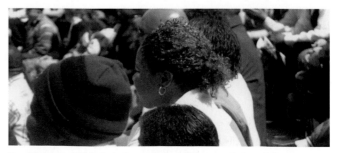

In Africa reddish hair is occasionally seen. It is not known whether this is an expression of gene pooling in the last 300 years after European immigration.

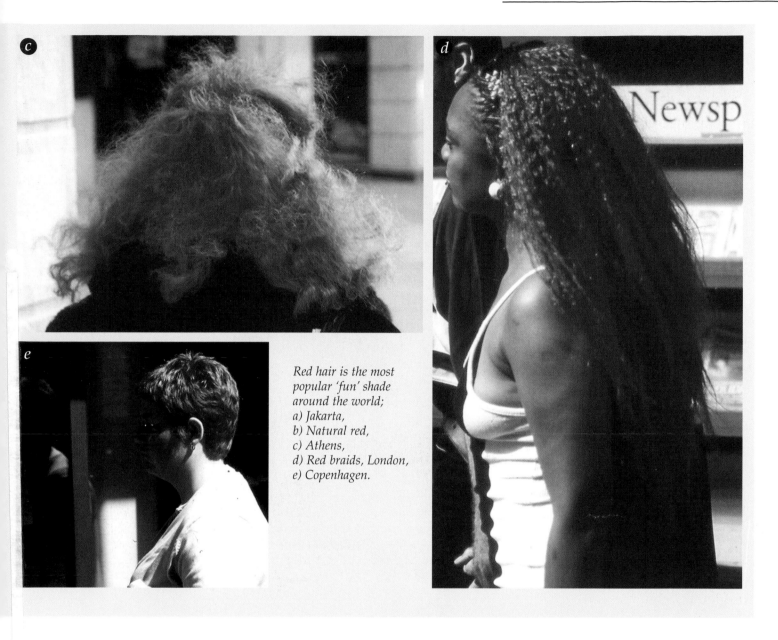

Red hair is the most
popular 'fun' shade
around the world;
a) Jakarta,
b) Natural red,
c) Athens,
d) Red braids, London,
e) Copenhagen.

SCIENCE BOX

It is suspected that red hair was able to emerge as a result of a mutation occurring in respect of a receptor gene in the hair follicle, which is activated through binding a sequence of amino-acids (peptide). It supports the manufacture of the most common and dark pigment, eumelanin.

This receptor can be inhibited by a special protein, the agouti signalling protein (ASP), and by mutation of tyrosine metabolism: the mutated pigment, phaeomelanin, gives lighter colours. This probably happened in the early history of humans in equatorial Africa,

although probably never in sufficient quantity to express in population terms. The view is that as humans migrated to more northern climes, natural selection constraints in Africa were removed or overcome, thus allowing what was essentially a rare mutation to emerge in large numbers.

People in northern Europe and their descendants who then migrated around the world to relatively uninhabited continents such as North America and Australasia are homozygous or compound heterozygotes for a few MC1R mutations.

Blondes

Pure natural 'blonde' is a very rare colour among the prevailing dark hair of most of humanity. It is not known when blonde hair emerged in human history but it has probably only appeared in the last few thousand years in any numbers. Unravelling the genetics of blonde hair has not been as easy as that for red hair. One major difficulty is the question of 'how blonde is blonde?' since there are many shades of blonde, including strawberry and ash blondes, plus the legion of the 'bleached blondes'.

Blonde hair, like red, almost certainly arose as a

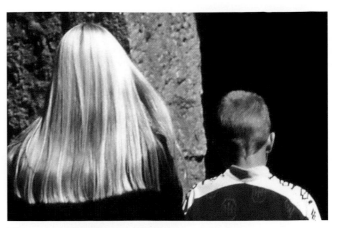

There are many shades of blonde.

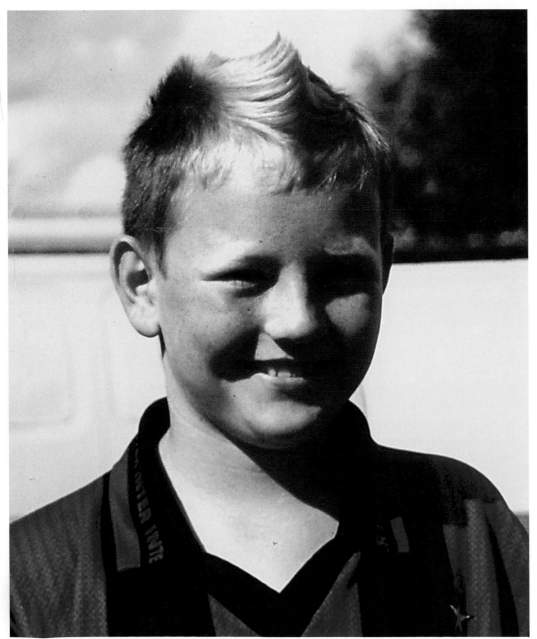

Even the very young try to emulate the appearance of their sporting icons!

late mutation of tyrosine metabolism and only survived in any numbers once early peoples had left Africa and probably as late as their arrival in Europe 35 000 years ago. We do not know the origin or time when truly light hair appeared, although mummies with blonde hair dating as far back as 2000 BC have been found in, surprisingly, China. It appears to have been spread throughout the southern Caucasus by 1000 BC.

The mode of inheritance of blonde hair is compatible with a recessive trait. It is still arguable whether blonde hair, like fair skin, is an evolutionary response to low levels of ultra-violet light in northern climes in order to maximize vitamin D production, since just 15 minutes exposure of an area the size of the forearm to ultra-violet light is all that is required for adequate vitamin production in humans. Whether the total body cover of early humans by hair, and their poorer overall nutrition for much of the year, played a part remains unknown.

Blonde hair is commoner in children than in adults, and may become less evident over time with the development of greater density of pigment, although exactly why this happens is not known.

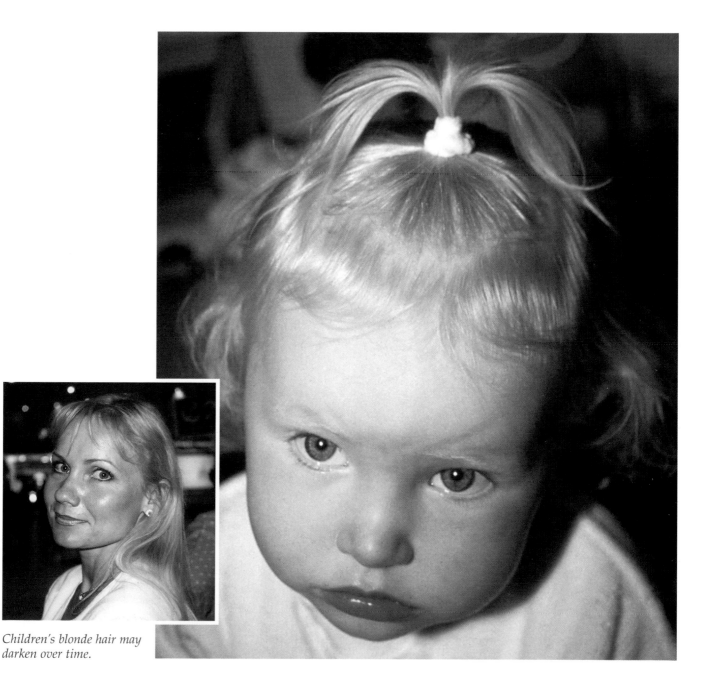

Children's blonde hair may darken over time.

Blondes in the 20th century

The rise of the ultra blonde has been meteoric, particularly since 1931 when the artificial platinum blonde Jean Harlow initiated a new phenomenon on screen. Hitherto 'vamps ' had been dark and sultry (viz., sexy). The blonde and sultry Harlow achieved fame at the same time as the rise of the political and economic liberation of women, particularly in the USA. Millions of women copied her, and the home and salon hair transformation business was born.

Two of the most charismatic women of the Western world, Marilyn Monroe and Diana Princess of Wales, rose to fame as luminescent 'blondes'.

Interestingly in the early 21st century blonde icons have been increasingly found more among sportsmen and women than straight movie stars. Anna Kournikova, Maria Sharpova and David Beckham are examples of individuals who through the power of the media and the ephemeral nature of blondeness, associated with youth and wholesomeness, have become global phenomena.

According to experts, at a basic psychological level blonde hair denotes youth. Mature women with a full head of naturally blonde hair are rare. The phenomenon of 'remembered blondeness' is a new concept.

HAIR MYTHS

Common misconceptions:

- blondes are less intelligent
- redheads are less serious
- brunettes are more trustworthy.

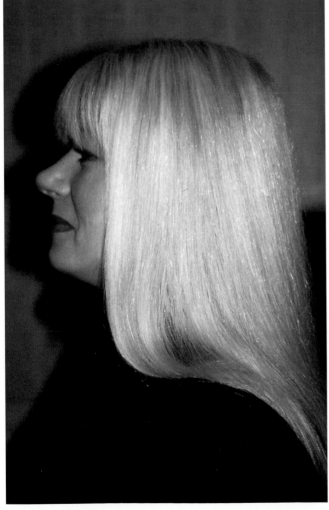

'Platinum' blonde.

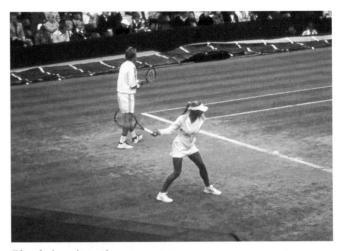

Blonde icon in action.

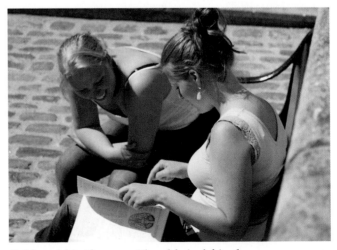

Golden girl in the sun with red-haired friend.

OPINIONS

A nationwide opinion survey in the USA found that:

- 60% of women in salons go blonde or highlight.
- 64% of all newscasters are blonde.
- 65% of all Miss Americas have been blonde.
- 62% of women see redheads as adventurous and daring.
- 82% of redheads see themselves as risk-takers compared to blondes (33%) and brunettes (19%).
- 83% of women agree that a brunette is better at managing money.
- 59% of women say a CEO would be likely to hire a brunette.
- 77% of women would trust a brunette with their deepest secret.

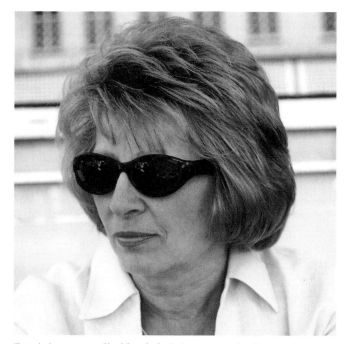

Retaining naturally blonde hair into maturity is rare.

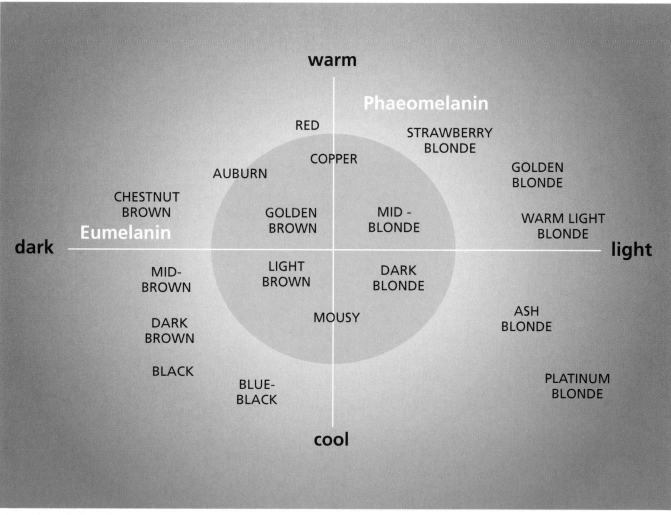

Natural tone/colour chart.

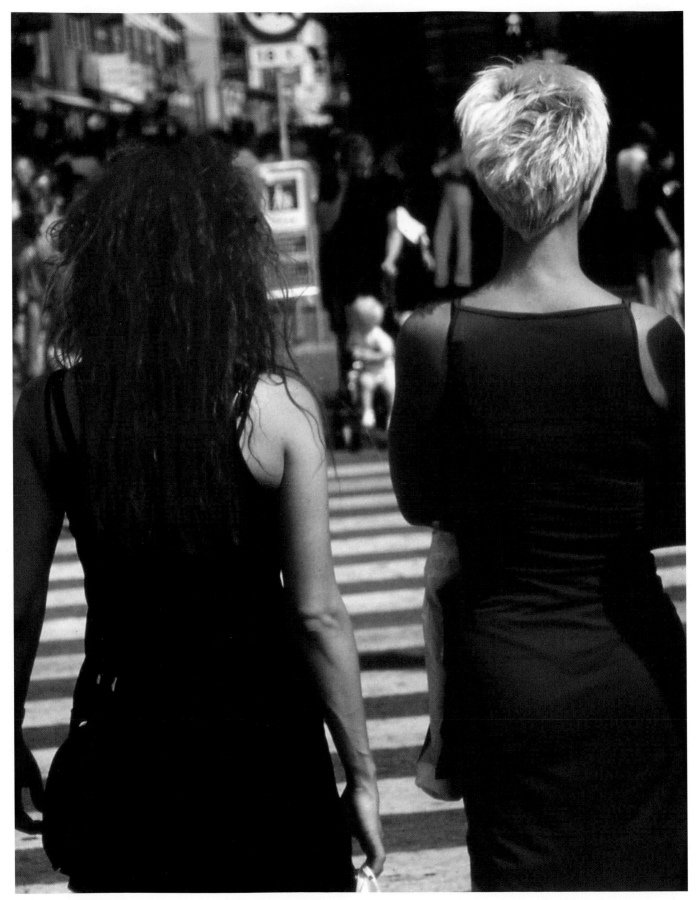

Two startling examples of hair colour wizardry.

5
Hair colour products

Our natural hair colour, like that of our eyes, is determined by complex sequences of genes and reflects millions of years of evolution, adaptation and convergence. Thanks to the development of hair dye products we can now, in minutes, create hair colour that may indeed be radically different from any natural human colour and circumvent evolution at a stroke.

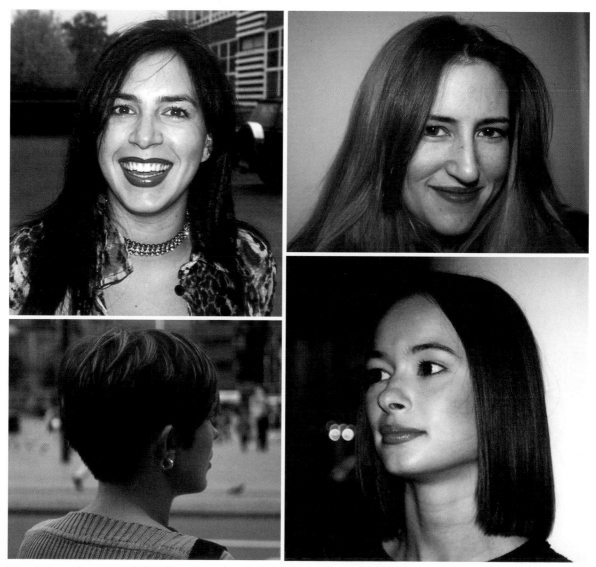

The ability to transform hair colour rapidly and safely reflects the almost magical skills of the cosmetic formulator.

The development of these products is not only based on the principles of good science and continuing research but follows fashion trends and the needs of the discerning hairdresser and consumer.

As a result bizarrely coloured apparently inert solutions are combined and then applied to the hair, resulting in hues to rival any the animal world can produce.

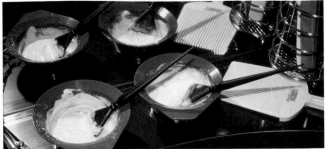

Hair dye solutions ready for use…

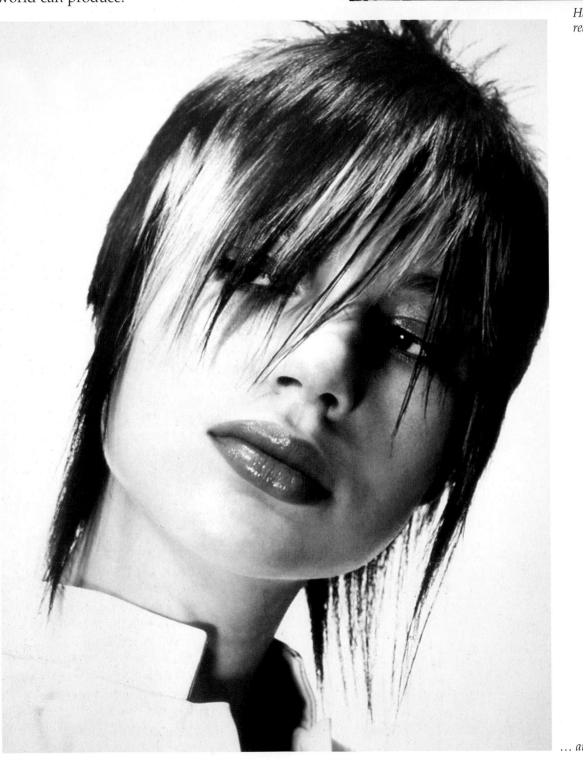

… and the result.

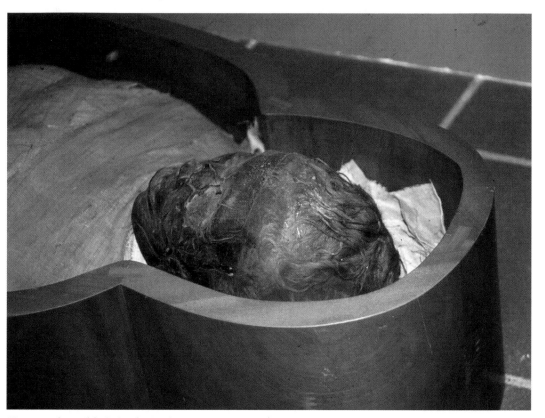

Henna-coloured hair in the Vatican Museums. An Egyptian mummy.

'Natural' ingredients such as henna and chamomile have been used throughout history: products containing only 'manufactured' ingredients, for just over 100 years. Whatever the eventual choice of the consumer, it is a combination of preference, convenience, reliability and safety that is important.

Inclusion of 'natural' ingredients in the manufactured range of products is now the practice of many of the top manufacturers, in response to strong consumer demand.

FACT BOX

Hair colour products are used by tens of millions of people and represent a business in excess of ten billion dollars annually.

Over six billion dollars of this is generated by self-purchase, and colouring accounts for almost half of the salon industry's revenue. Over 70% of women in the developed world have coloured their hair at least once, and 30% do so every six weeks. In China it is now estimated that 40% of women are using such products.

In this chapter we examine the role of hair colouring in history through to the present day. We explore the extraordinary skills of colour chemistry and offer some insights into how to achieve that perfect transformation.

Artificial hair colour throughout history

The earliest known depictions of humans are figures in the 40 000-year-old cave paintings of France, followed much later by Middle Eastern tomb and palace drawings, which show darkly pigmented hair. In Egyptian hieroglyphics dark-haired royalties were probably depicted as wearing wigs, although whether these were made from human hair is not known.

Kohl and henna were used as artificial pigments in cosmetics in Egyptian times, and Cleopatra is reputed to have used both (mimicked Hollywood-style by Elizabeth Taylor).

The ancients had neither the theoretical chemistry of modern scientists, nor any access to their technical armamentarium. Lightening the hair often depended on the application of hideous mixtures of crude chemicals and natural excretion products. The Grecian sect of Aphrodite (depicted by a blonde goddess of Athens) used mixtures of potash to lighten their hair. Athenian courtesans bleached their hair as a mark of their profession.

Roman women, possibly envying their light-haired slaves and wishing to mimic them, employed a mixture of 'natural' products such as wood ash, unslaked lime (quicklime) and sodium bicarbonate, wild fruits and alcohol. These, when left in the hair over several days and exposed to the sunlight, are reported to have had a bleaching effect. Less affluent aficionados used bird dung and horse urine

(there is no record of the aroma or of its marketing success). Other reported and equally vile mixtures include a fermented composite of leeches and animal urine.

Copper solutions were used for darker shades: the toxicity of some of these preparations must have been truly formidable.

The widespread use of plant extracts such as henna developed in Asia as a way of producing a lighter shade on essentially dark hair. Its use persists to this day, and it has been carried from its homeland to other countries where it remains the mainstay of colour transformation (see page 78).

For over 100 years, in Restoration times and in post-Revolutionary France, a combination of an

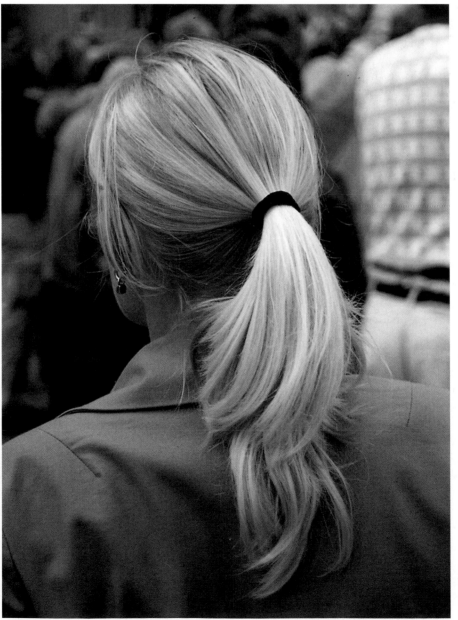

Modern lightening products avoid the toxicity of previous centuries.

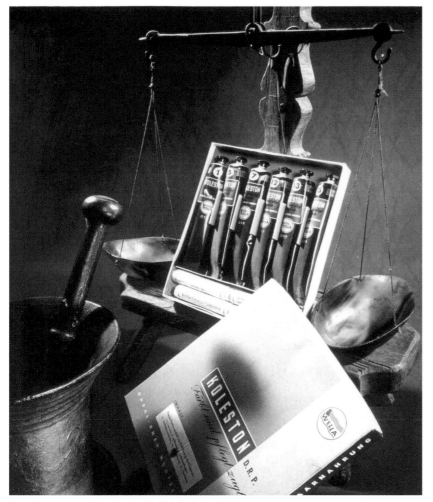

The first cream permanent colours from Wella.

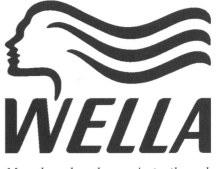

Many logos have become instantly, and internationally, recognizable.

alkaline salt and the sun was popular. Caustic soda or wood ash (which contains another caustic, potassium hydroxide) were widely used – an example of the unwitting use of oxidative chemistry. Again, in the sophisticated society of Napoleonic Paris, potassium hydroxide became fashionable for lightening hair. It can only be imagined that the time and effort involved reflected an age less obsessed with time or product liability.

The late 19th century saw the breakthrough in chemistry that led to the birth of the hair dye industry (see below). As the 20th century progressed the art and science of colour chemistry advanced, and in tandem with mass media, particularly the cinema, exposed the 'masses' to new icons and new aspirations. The scale of copying of hair style and colour reached worldwide proportions.

The introduction of mass market and salon hair dyes in any great volume in the 20th

century by companies such as Clairol and Wella brought about a global revolution and an explosion of colouring available to huge numbers of consumers.

The story began in 1863, when the legendary chemist Dr Hofmann reported the dye properties of a substance that has since come to dominate the field of permanent hair colouring, *para*-phenylenediamine (usually abbreviated to *p*-phenylenediamine, or PPD). The original patent stated that hair could be 'dyed brown by immersion in a solution of the diamine and hydrogen peroxide'.

Dr Hofmann's discovery still dominates the hair dye market, as permanent dyes derived from PPD account for over 70% of all products sold. This process of dyeing might be more accurately described as 'staining', since significant amounts of dyes are rinsed away during the process.

The early years of hair colorants were not without controversy, as witnessed by the

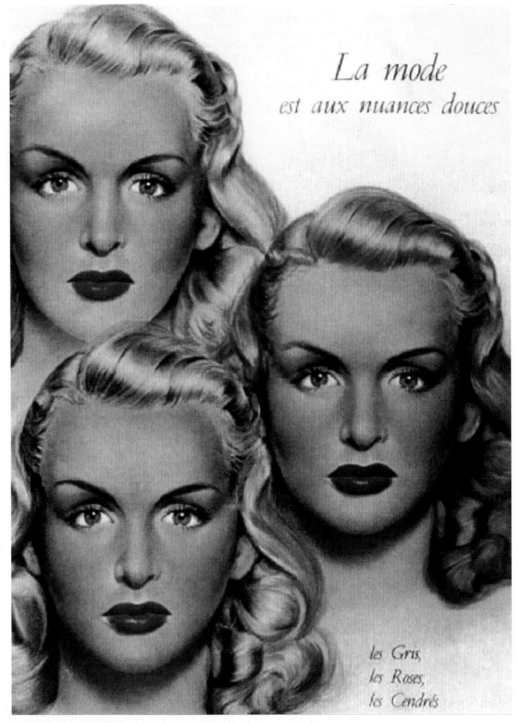

La mode
est aux nuances douces

les Gris,
les Roses,
les Cendrés

Early Clairol advert showing 'transformation'.

uncompromising comment in *Ladies' Home Journal* in 1892: 'It goes without saying that a well-bred woman does not dye her hair.' Even in the years following World War I, hair dyeing could still be problematic.

The real breakthrough came when Clairol launched their first home colours in 1931 and millions of women used them, particularly in imitation of Jean Harlow. Development continued throughout the next 20 years, with the legendary advertising copy 'has she or hasn't she?' and 'is she or isn't she?' epitomizing the excitement these products could bring.

In 1953 Wella launched the first crème permanent dyes and transformed the hair colouring business.

Modern hair dyes

Modern international manufacturers of hair dye products have established some of the most sophisticated research and development organizations in order to develop new hair colour products. They work extensively with a close group of expert hairdressers and hair technicians both internally and externally, to ensure that use in the salon and the home meets technical needs as well as those of consumers. Moreover, they acquire deep understanding of consumer attitudes and needs, and follow fashion trends and fashion icons in the never-ending quest to produce products that appeal to the uninitiated. This process is supported by some of the best research chemists and formulators of hair dye products in the world, whose skills are similar to those of expert wine and tea tasters in their ability to detect subtle differences in shade and, more especially, in tones.

They look for subtle shades that will not 'go brassy' or 'fade', that can be used by millions of people with regular and reliable results, and that meet all the quality and safety criteria dictated by regulations and commercial success. The following is an example of the development process:

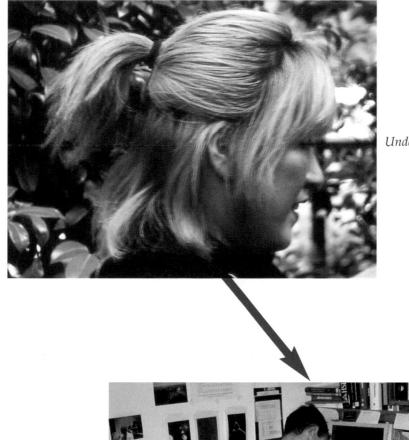

Understanding consumer needs.

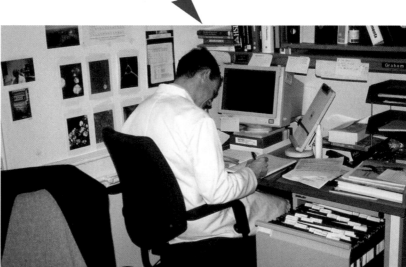

Products research – defining the 'new' shade.

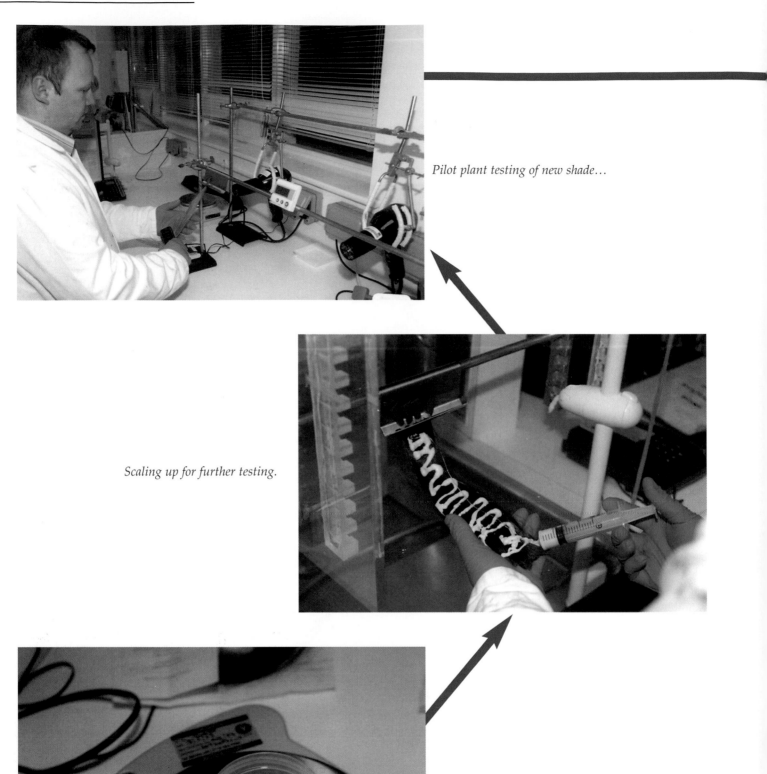

Pilot plant testing of new shade…

Scaling up for further testing.

Selection of 'couplers' and lab formulation. Testing will be on hair swatches and in the salon.

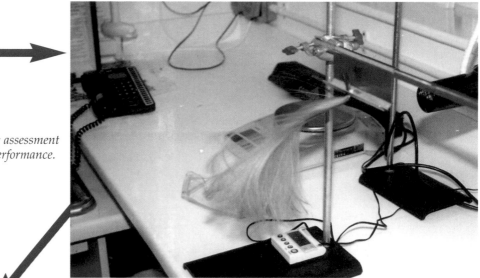

... including assessment of product performance.

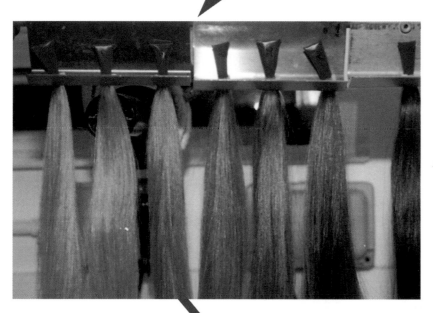

A range of shades...

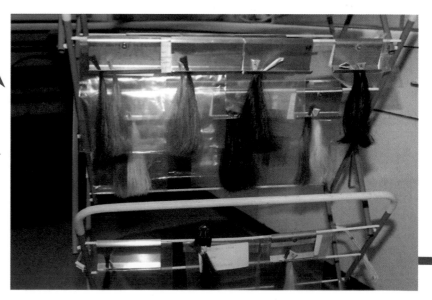

... from the lightest to the darkest.

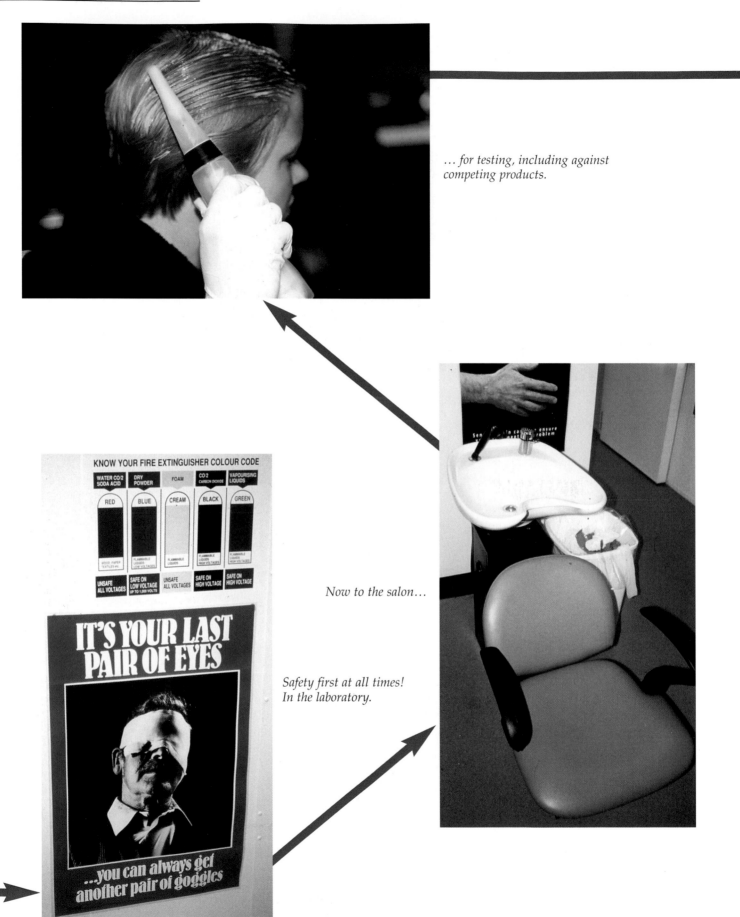

… for testing, including against competing products.

Now to the salon…

*Safety first at all times!
In the laboratory.*

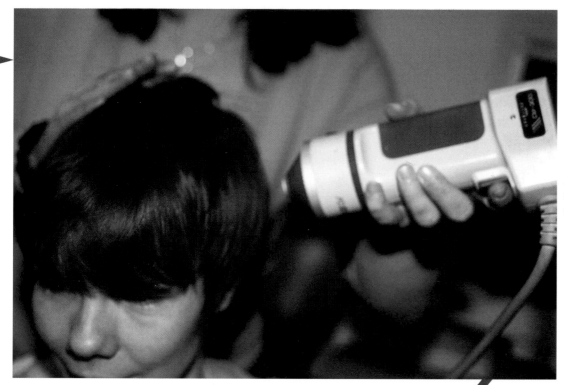

Assessing the colour results with a reflectometer...

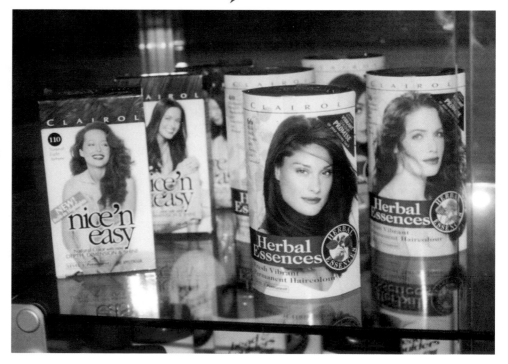

... and finally, in the market place.

Each of these stages will have feedback to the previous step, and the product may require reformulation at any stage.

For simplicity, *modern hair dyes* can be divided into four basic categories:

- temporary
- semi-permanent
- permanent
- other dyes.

Temporary colorants are water-soluble acid or high-molecular-weight ionic basic dyes, which coat the outside of the hair shaft, and which under normal conditions do not penetrate the cuticle and so are easily removed at the first shampooing (see page 67).

A second class of temporary colorants are basic dyes with large cationic molecules having some attraction for the hair and consequently better fastness, but which are still deposited only on the hair surface.

Temporary dyes may be an excellent place to start colour transformation, allowing the user to see what works and what does not. A disaster is easily rectified.

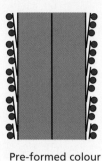
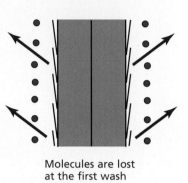

Pre-formed colour complexes singly coat the cuticle

Molecules are lost at the first wash

Temporary colorants: how they work.

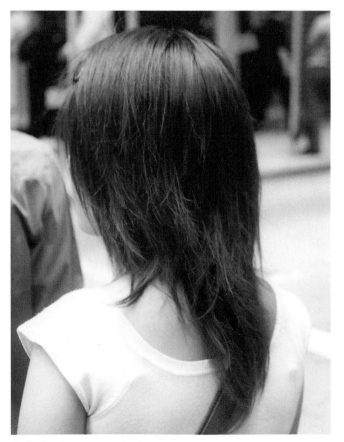

A daring transformation!

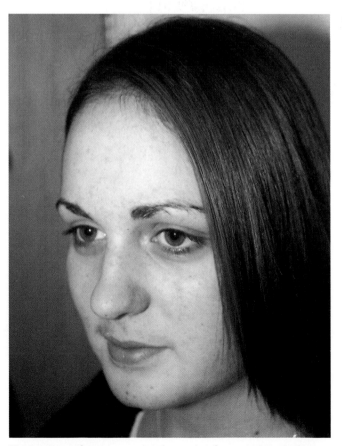

Temporary colorants – a starting-point for experimentation.

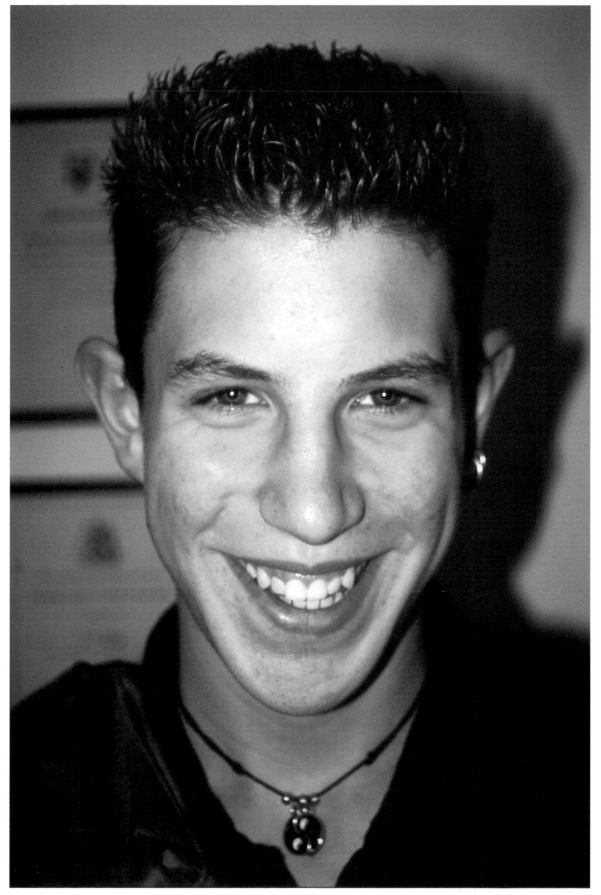

Temporary dyes may be an excellent place to start colour transformation to see what works and what does not.

Semi-permanent products use low-molecular-weight ingredients such as nitroaromatic amines or aromatic dyes which do penetrate into the fibre to produce the colour effect. Since they are not exposed to oxidation, however, they are not bound to the hair protein and can be washed out, over typically between four and six wash cycles. Semi-permanent dyes can make the hair the same depth of colour as the natural base or darker, but they cannot lighten hair. They are referred to as **Level 1 products** by cosmetic companies.

Permanent dyes are (almost) literally that – they cannot be washed out, and only slowly fade from oxidation with ultra-violet light. Their success and popularity is due to their extreme versatility, and some 80% of hair colorants used fall in this category.

Shades lighter or darker than the base colour can be achieved.

Level 2 products developed in the last ten years have little or no lightening potential and less thorough grey coverage, but a shorter dyeing time. They are useful when grey is less than 20% of the hair colour.

Level 3 products have the longest-lasting and most complete grey coverage, but require longer application time. The effects these products achieve can be spectacular: striking blondes and vibrant reds, or subtle mid-browns for grey coverage.

The main difference between Level 2 and Level 3 products is the alkalizing agent and the concentration of peroxide. Level 3 products usually employ ammonia and up to 6% hydrogen peroxide, compared with only 3% peroxide together with a non-ammonia alkalizer (monoethanolamine, for instance) for Level 2 products.

Other dyes include metallic dyes and vegetable dyes (see page 78).

SCIENCE BOX

Each of the 150 000 hairs on our heads may be the target for temporary, semi-permanent or permanent hair dyes. The state of the hair – known by hair scientists as the **substrate** – may affect the outcome.

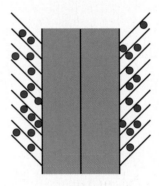

Pre-formed colour complexes penetrate cuticle scales and deposit (helped by warming action in plastic cap provided)

Colour complexes become trapped under cuticle scales which slightly open during the warming action

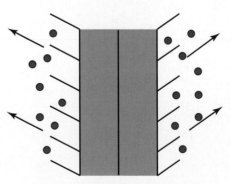

Colour is released slowly over 6–8 shampoos (depending on hair porosity) as complexes have not penetrated deep into hair cortex (see page 67)

Level 1 colorants – how do they work?

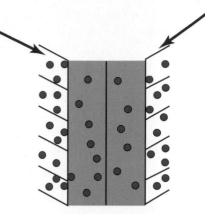

Small building blocks easily diffuse through hair cortex where developer lightens natural colour and assemble colour into larger complexes

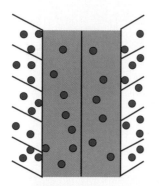

Small building blocks easily diffuse through hair cortex where the colour is developed by oxygen (low level of developer – no ammonia)

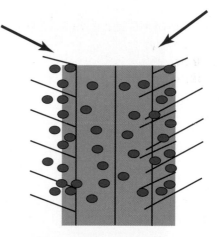

Colour building blocks diffuse into hair cortex thanks to ammonia. Hair is slightly 'swollen' – this dramatically helps colour diffusion

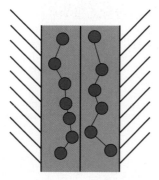

Oxidation forms large colour complexes so that developed colour is trapped within the hair fibre in the cortex. Penetration is less efficient than with Level 3 permanent colorants, due to lack of ammonia swelling effect

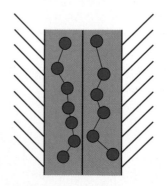

A permanent complex is formed throughout hair cortex, so colour is virtually permanent – mimicking natural melanin granules

Level 2 colorants – how do they work?

Level 3 colorants – how do they work?

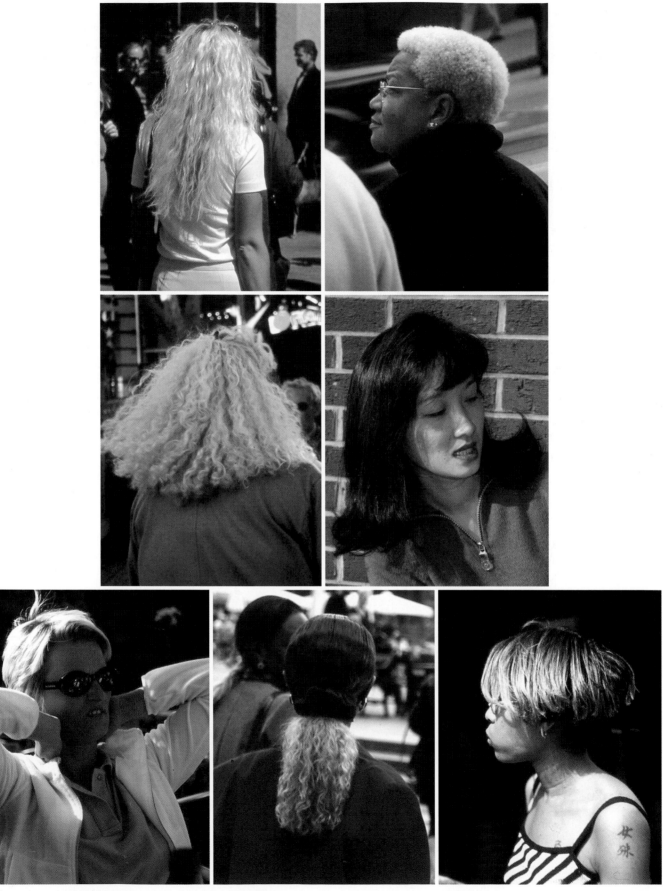

Fabulous use of bleaching chemistry around the world.

Permanent hair dyeing

Physically hair is composed of proteins (keratin) embedded in a sulphur-rich matrix encased in an even richer sheath of overlapping scales. There are three main physical components of the hair:

- The **cuticle** consists of 5–10 layers of overlapping scales, which protect the hair and

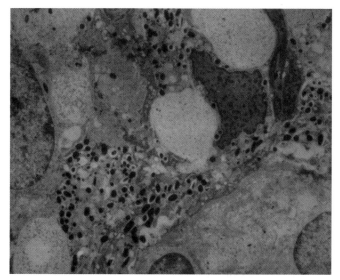

Electronmicrograph of a single hair shaft showing the dense pigment-bearing cortex and the outer cuticle.

give it its 'sensory' properties when you run your hands through it. Each scale is 0.5–1 μ thick and around 45 μ long. The cuticle acts as a physical and chemical barrier to dye diffusion.

- The **cortex** makes up the bulk of the hair and is composed of keratin (a sulphur rich protein). It is here that most melanin is found, primarily at the periphery.

- The **medulla** is a soft proteinaceous core not found in most pigmented hairs but more common in grey hairs. It is not involved in the dyeing process.

Permanent hair dyeing can generate a range of colours, from the straightforward to the exotic. The process is both apparently simple and yet complex from a chemical standpoint.

Permanent hair dyes contain **precursors**, which are essential ingredients common to most permanent dyes. Normally these are substances called *p*-diamines and *p*-aminophenols.

These precursors are oxidized by hydrogen peroxide to **active intermediates** once they have penetrated into the hair shaft. These intermediates then react (within the hair shaft) with additional ingredients in the product – **colour couplers** – to give wash-resistant dyes.

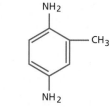

p-Phenylenediamine

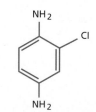

Toluene-2,5-diamine

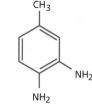

Toluene-3,4-diamine

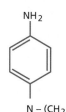

N,N-Bis(2-hydroxyethyl)-p-phenylenediamine

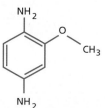

2-Methoxy-p-phenylenediamine

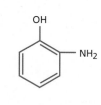

2-Chloro-p-phenylenediamine

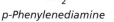

o-Aminophenol

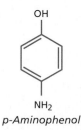

p-Aminophenol

Some oxidation dye precursors.

[*Source* P & G data on file]

Oxidation dye couplers are electron-rich aromatics:

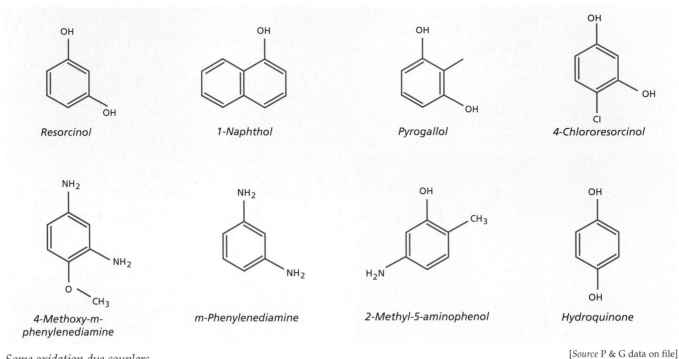

Some oxidation dye couplers.

[Source P & G data on file]

Precursors themselves form grey or black-brown compounds in the presence of hydrogen peroxide. This is why they are important in darker shades, particularly for covering grey hair. Couplers do not themselves produce colour but modify the colour produced by the oxidation of precursor compounds. In more complex colours the products may contain several precursors and many couplers, and involve very many reactions after penetrating the hair. The colour imparted to the hair relies on the ratio of the various intermediates used and on their total concentration.

Shade formulation is very complicated. Colours of common coupler/precursor combinations are determined by the skilled formulator. The 'alchemy' lies in the ability to formulate the desired shade with the correct level of vibrancy and to prevent fading 'off-shade' (i.e. going 'brassy') after a few washes. Formulators will assess the result on hair swatches and can by the addition or deletion of couplers effect the desired change.

Table of developers and couplers used in a typical hair colour range	
Developers	**Couplers**
p-Phenylenediamine	m-Phenylenediamine sulphate
p-Aminophenol	Resorcinol (RS)
o-Aminophenol	1-Naphthol
Diaminotoluene sulphate	4-Amino-2-hydroxytoluene
N,N-bis(hydroxyethyl)-p-PD sulphate	2-Amino-3-hydroxypyridine
p-Methylaminophenol	m-Aminophenol
	2-Methylresorcinol
	2-Methyl-5-hydroxyethylaminophenol
	2-Amino-4-hydroxyethylaminoanisole sulphate

SCIENCE BOX

Three steps to colour

- The primary intermediates are usually derivatives of either *p*-phenylenediamine (PPD) or of *p*-aminophenol.
- PPD and its derivatives are the intermediates responsible for dark brown and black shades.
- *p*-Aminophenol is responsible for light auburn and its derivatives for pale blondes.

Step 1
Primary intermediates are oxidized by hydrogen peroxide and must be capable of forming a quinoid structure (such as those of 1,4-diketones and their derivatives – the active colouring material of henna, see page 78, is an example). When precursors are oxidized in isolation they form coloured compounds, usually grey or brown-black.

Step 2
The oxidized primary intermediate then reacts with another aromatic molecule, the coupler, at the most nucleophilic carbon atom on the structure.

Step 3
This coupled reaction product is oxidized to the final coloured dye molecule. These dimers can go on to form trimers, tetramers and so forth. These bulky reaction products have low water solubility; both of these factors help to make the product wash- and fade-resistant.

The colour imparted to the hair relies on the ratio of the various intermediates used and on their total concentration.

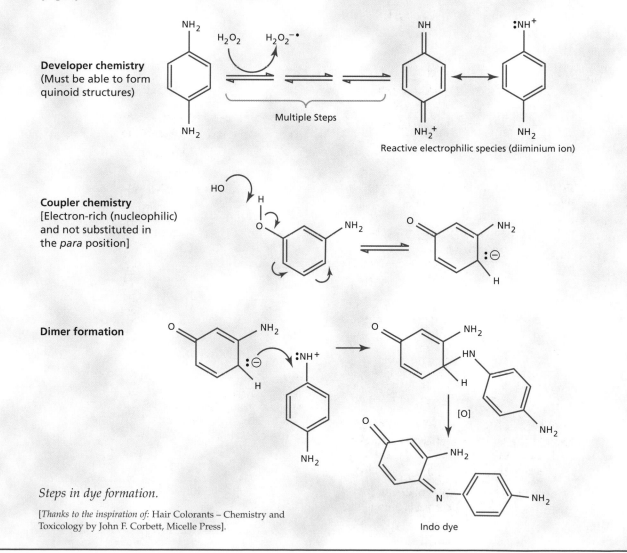

Steps in dye formation.

[*Thanks to the inspiration of*: Hair Colorants – Chemistry and Toxicology by John F. Corbett, Micelle Press].

Active ingredients (other than dyes) in the colorant base

Ammonia: When hair is treated with hydrogen peroxide alone almost no bleaching is observed. To get the lightening, an alkalizer is needed to activate the system, the most effective one being ammonia. The ingredient ammonium persulphate is one of the most commonly used.

The levels of ammonia and peroxide added will determine how much bleaching occurs; for blonde shades, more is added than for darker shades. More is not always better, however, as too much ammonia irritates the scalp and makes the product smell even worse than normal. The addition of ammonia also raises the pH of the product to around 10; at this pH hair swells, allowing the dye materials mentioned above to penetrate further into the hair. Once in the hair the dye reactions take place, giving rise to wash-fast and fade-resistant colours.

Chelants: Peroxide is inherently unstable. Without ingredients that bind metals present in the product or water and in a low pH, the activity of the peroxide would rapidly be lost. The role of the chelants is to deactivate any trace amounts of catalytic metals that may get into the product. This deactivation of the metals occurs by two mechanisms:

- altering the redox potential of the metal so that it is less prone to undergo catalytic redox cycles

- strongly binding to the metal at all the available reaction sites; the most important are those for iron and copper.

In an ideal world, zero contamination of products or the environment by metals would be desirable. In practice, however, minute quantities (measured in parts per billion), which are impossible to remove, will cause unstabilized peroxide to decompose.

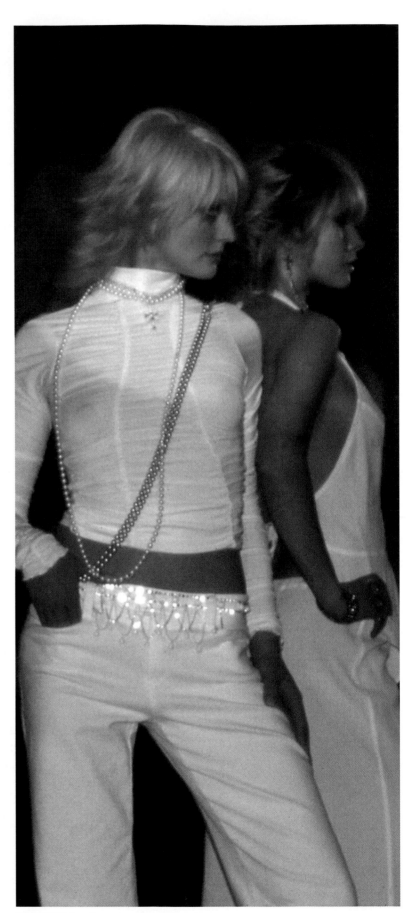

Hair 'lift' for the catwalk.

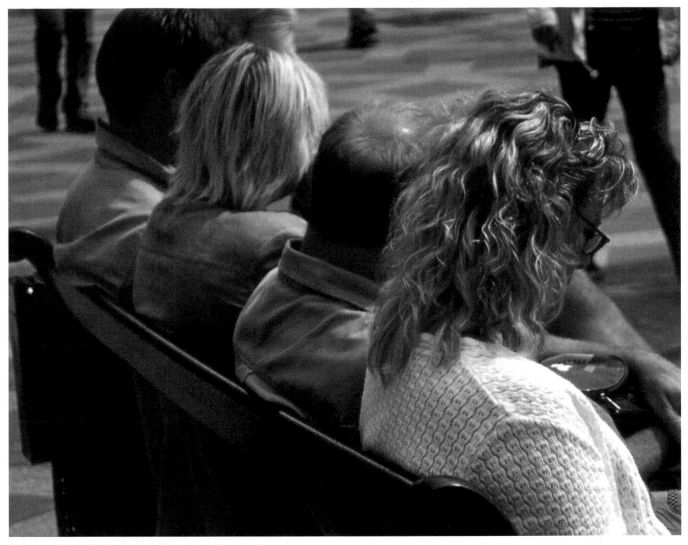

The use of hair lightening products is widespread.

Consequently, great care must be taken in manufacture and packing to prevent any contamination of the peroxide base. To minimize peroxide loss a chelant system is added to the peroxide; this prevents trace metals from catalysing the decomposition of the peroxide.

Solvents: These are added for two reasons:

■ to solubilize the dye materials, which in general dissolve in water only with difficulty, and

■ to help improve viscosity and flow properties by working with the surfactant system.

It is important to get the dyes into solution at the lowest possible temperature, in order to reduce the amount of oxidation to a minimum, to stop the solution from discolouring and to maintain the dye concentration. Currently used solvents include dipropylene glycol, hexylene glycol, ethanol and glycerin.

Surfactants/fatty alcohols: These materials have several roles in the product. Primarily they act as viscosity modifiers giving pack compatibility and reducing mess during, and after, application. The ceteareth-25 and steareth-2 are emulsifiers that hold the entire system together, and they also help to remove oil and sebum from the hair surface giving even dyeing. Addition of cetyl and stearyl alcohol helps both conditioning and flow properties.compatible with the applicator and reduce drip in use.

An alternative to a cream product is one that uses two thin liquids that thicken on mixing. This system allows easy mixing of the peroxide and dye phases. Both cream and liquid systems are common in the market place.

Hydrogen peroxide: Hydrogen peroxide is used in colour transformation to provide oxygen to 'fuel' the reactions. Without it, no permanent colour would be formed.

The peroxide base functions are:

- to activate the colorant chemistry by oxidizing the dye species
- to bleach out the colour of hair (melanin and residual dyes), allowing the desired shade to be achieved.

Typical peroxide levels are 3% and 4.5% 'on head'.

The colour transformation

Psychological aspects

The decision to effect a transformation of hair colour is a 'moment of truth'. There are many personal, psychological and practical aspects to consider.

A commonly cited reason is simply despair at one's natural colour. In the teenage years, mid-brown or 'mouse' colour seem to provoke an overwhelming desire to change. A colour change may be dictated by fashion, by a celebrity icon, or the single most common reason – covering grey.

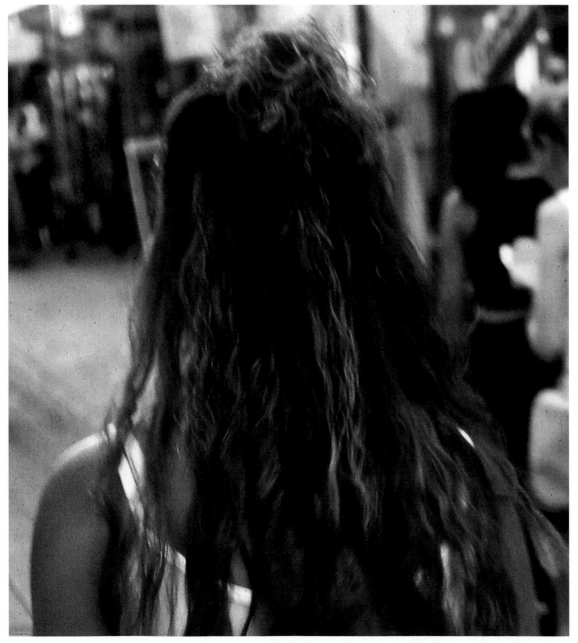

Once embarked upon a radical change it may be difficult to go back.

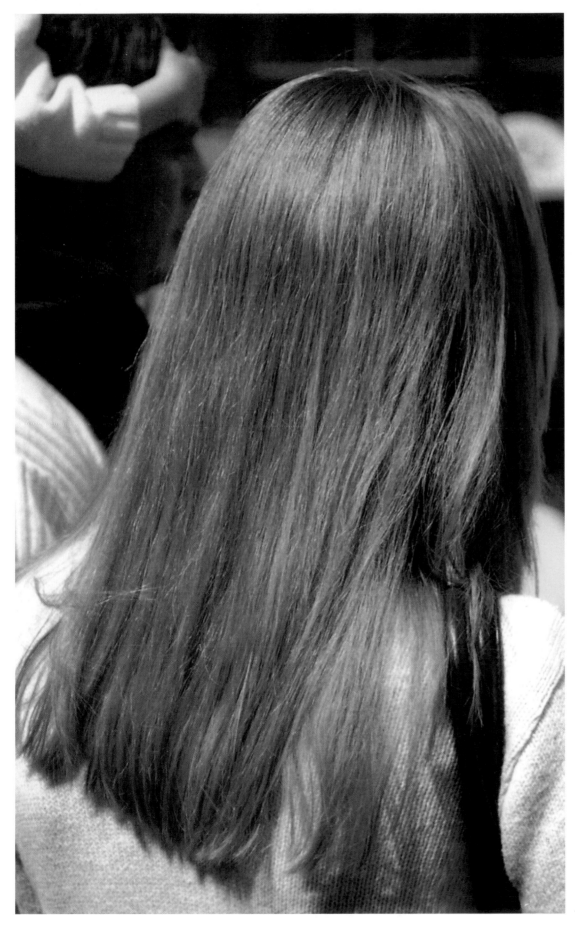

In the teenage years, mid-brown or 'mouse' hair colour often provokes an overwhelming desire for dramatic change.

Those who regularly cover their grey hairs may feel 'naked' if they fail to do so, and once started it may be very difficult to stop. Those who feel that grey is just 'part of nature's rich pattern' should not despise those in whom it engenders pathological dismay.

Changing colour may be part of an attempt to change one's image or life. Lightening hair after a divorce or on emerging from bereavement is common; a lifting depression is often accompanied by a vibrant colour transformation. These are the 'inner' and 'outer' motivators.

For most of us, however, departing too far from nature's intent may send a harsher message than working from the original base range. Working with what Mother Nature has given,

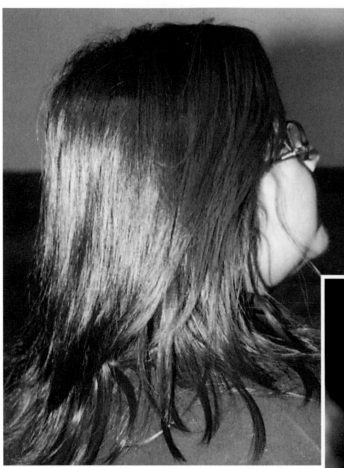

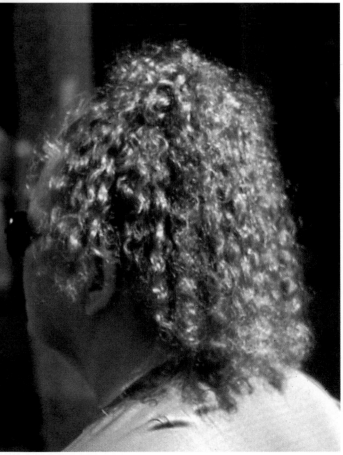

Departing too far from nature's intent may send a harsh message.

understanding the science of hair colouring and taking care of hair afterwards are the keynotes to success.

A recent UK survey conducted by a leading hair colorant company found that two-thirds of women colour their hair simply to change their appearance. Sometimes they aim to look like their favourite female celebrity, while an amazing 90% of women feel that colour can impact their ability to climb up the corporate ladder!

A striking majority, 77%, of women use an alteration in their hair colour as a vital way of boosting confidence and 49% felt 'sexier' having made the change.

Brunettes are viewed as 'practical' and as having the most likely colouring for the first

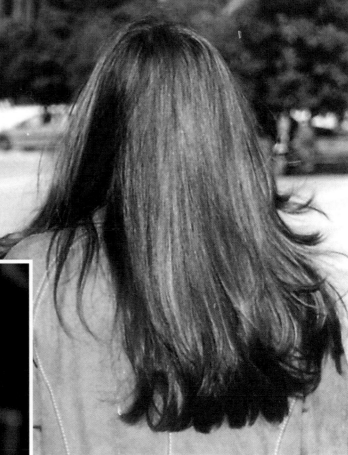

Exploiting Mother Nature's gifts, together with the alchemy of hair colouring followed by meticulous hair care, are the keynotes to success.

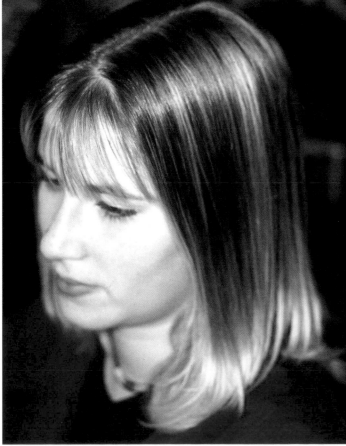

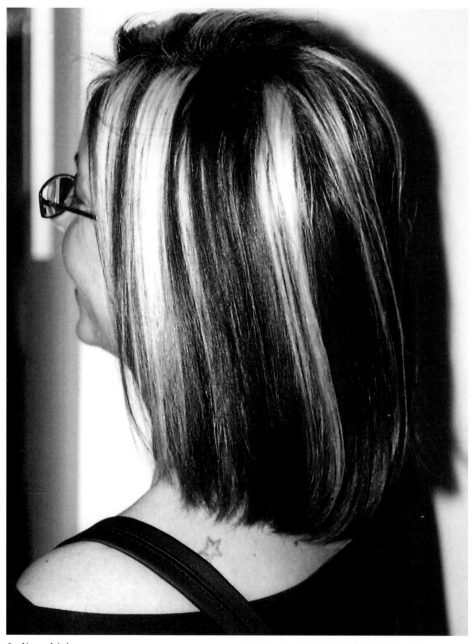

Italian chic!

female President of the USA. They are thought to have the 'best' family life but to be the most likely to have verbal disagreements.

Blondes are viewed as glamorous, wealthy and pampered. They are 'head-turners', but are reported to have poorer love lives than brunettes or redheads.

Redheads are seen as risk-takers with 'good sex lives'. Over half the women interviewed said they would like to become a redhead for the day – but most thought that redheads would be the least likely to be offered a top job.

An overwhelming 86% felt heads of government should *not* cover their grey hair as this conveys an impression of wisdom.

Welsh ladies appear to be the true chameleons of hair colour, with a significant 88% stating that they colour their hair in order to achieve a 'transformation'. Similarly, Welsh women seem to be the most modern in their approach to men colouring their hair, with 81% supportive. Across the UK, however, an average of 34% of women feel that a man who dyes his hair is 'vain'.

Two-thirds of women change their hair colour to realize their fantasies, whether at work or at play.

How to choose the right shade

Remember that the colour of the model's hair on the front of the box is only a guide to the final colour result. To see what *your* hair will look like, check the back of the box where swatches show the result of applying the particular product. And bear in mind the 'golden rule' of hair colouring:

Natural Hair Colour + Shade used = Final colour result.

FANTASY MYTHS EXPLODED

A colour survey included a question as to whether gentlemen really prefer blondes – and do women care?

81% of women said that men fantasize most about blondes, but when asked about their own fantasy hair colour their response was an emphatic anti-blonde!

HAIR COLOUR DEPTHS AND TONES

Hair colorants come in different depths – light, medium or dark. Every hair colour is also available in warm tones (warm and golden shades), cool tones (ash shades) or a balance (neutral or natural shades). These unique tones add a special dimension to your hair colour.

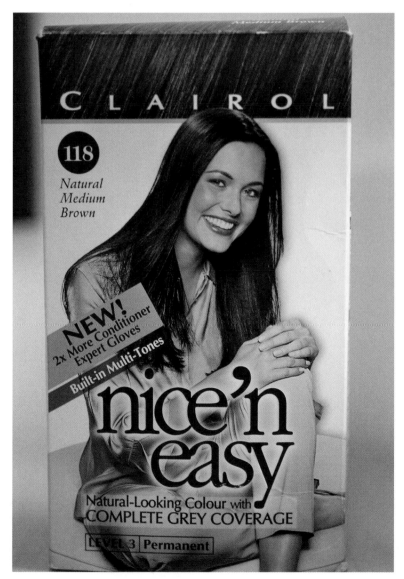

Modern permanent hair dye packaging.

Natural and vegetable colouring agents

Since the earliest times, natural organic substances have been gathered from plants and used as hair dyes. Two substances stand out: henna and camomile.

Henna is probably the most famous 'natural' hair colorant in the world. It was certainly used in Egypt thousands of years ago to colour the hair red – it is still extensively used in Asia and by Asian peoples in the West.

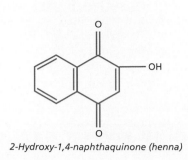

2-Hydroxy-1,4-naphthaquinone (henna)

The active colouring material of henna.

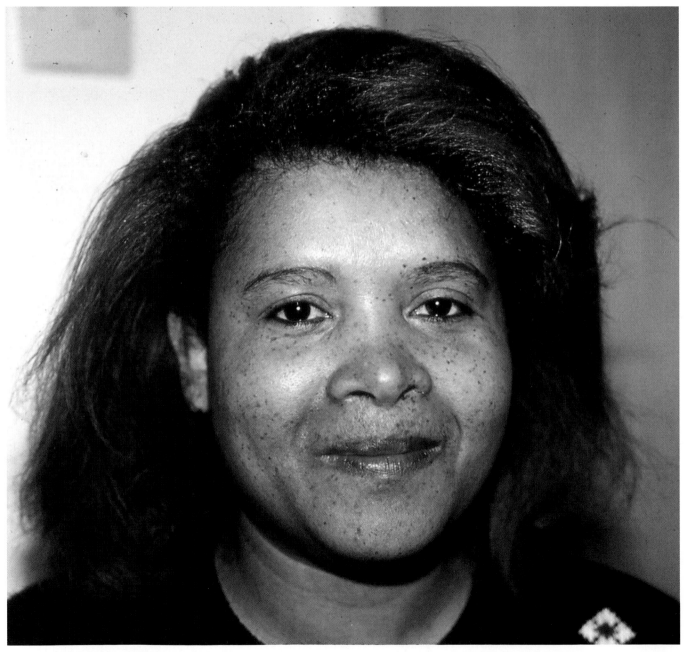

Typical hennaed hair – Malaysia.

Henna is a temporary dye which covers the outer surface of the hair shaft. It is derived from the crushed, dried leaves of the Egyptian privet (*Lawsonia alba*), which grows in Asia and northern Africa. The active ingredient is lawsone, isolated in 1709 by the famous botanist Dr Israel Lawson. The leaves are harvested, sun-dried, crushed into a green powder and extracted with aqueous sodium bicarbonate. The tone produced on the hair depends on the time of gathering, and if the leaves are not fully mature a delicate shade of red with a slight yellow tone is given. Fully mature henna gives a deeper red: thus the colour produced is not absolutely predictable. It is also mixed with a variety of other herbs such as camomile, sage or indigo, which gives Persian henna – a deep blue-black. Many women mix the powder with tea or coffee before applying.

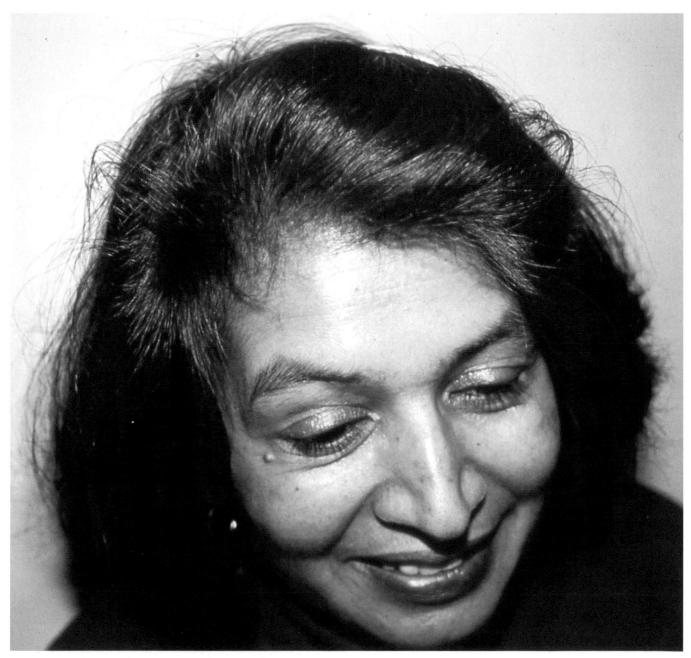

India – this lady mixes henna with coffee before applying.

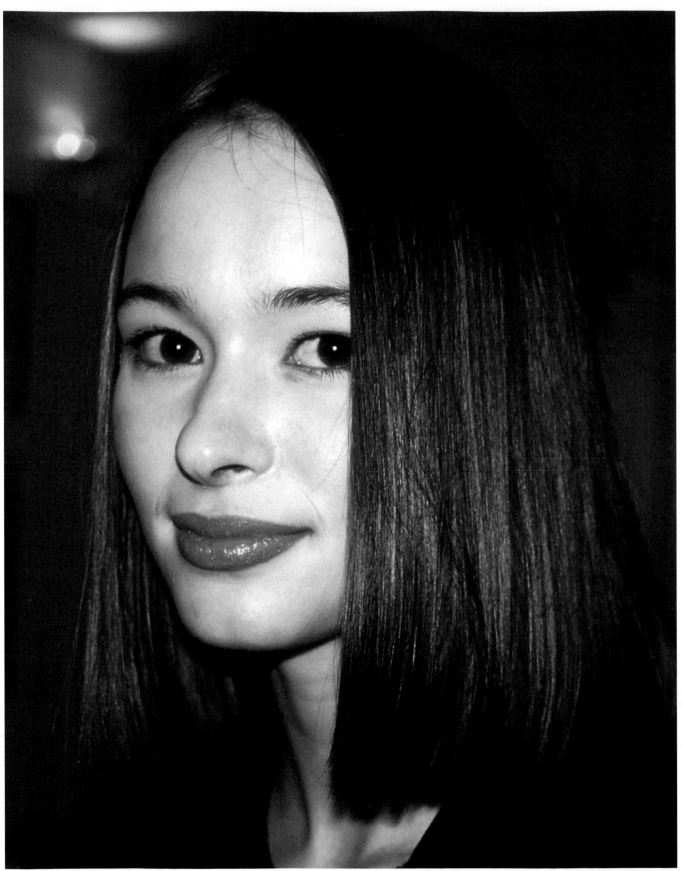

Subtle tones – professional excellence.

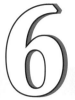

Colouring hair: scientific and practical aspects

Actual on-head colours

There are so many gorgeous shades, it is difficult for a beginner to know which one to choose.

The glamorous picture on the box is just that – the colour on the model. It is important to choose from the shade selector grid – this gives an approximate indication of the final colour the user can expect, starting from the natural hair colour.

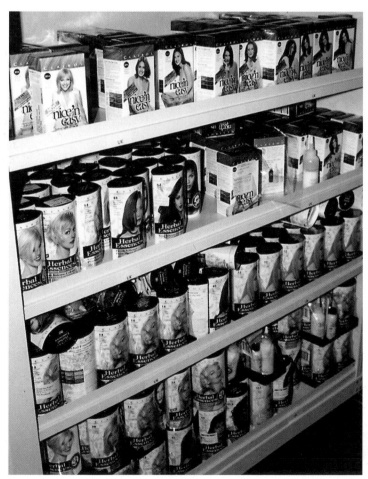

It's hard to choose from the range of wonderful shades.

The natural or base colour will be determined by the relative proportions of eumelanin and phaeomelanin, together with the percentage of grey hair present. It is easy to forget that from about 20 onwards every head carries the occasional grey hair. By the age of 50 this may be up to 50% of total hairs.

The final shade depends on certain major factors other than the combination of dyes:

1. The initial colour of the hair: The darker the starting material, the harder it is to get to a blonde. Moreover, hair that has a distinct root line is more difficult to colour evenly.

2. The condition of the hair: Damaged hair is more porous than virgin hair, and acts like a sponge. It easily absorbs dyes, darkening faster than the less absorbent undamaged hair. This open nature of damaged hair also facilitates more rapid colour washout.

Aftercare, with intense moisturizing, is crucial.

3. The hair type: The physical dimensions of the hair are relevant – Oriental hair tends to be thicker and requires greater volume of dye than fine Nordic hair.

4. The time the product is on the hair: The longer the product is on the hair the more colour is formed and the more the natural shade is bleached.

5. Other colour considerations
   - The colour of the skin and eyebrows may play an important part in the aesthetic success of a transformation. Light skin and blue eyes naturally complement blonde hair. Occasionally blue eyes occur naturally with dark hair, but a combination of red hair and dark skin is a radical departure that may be a challenge to look natural.

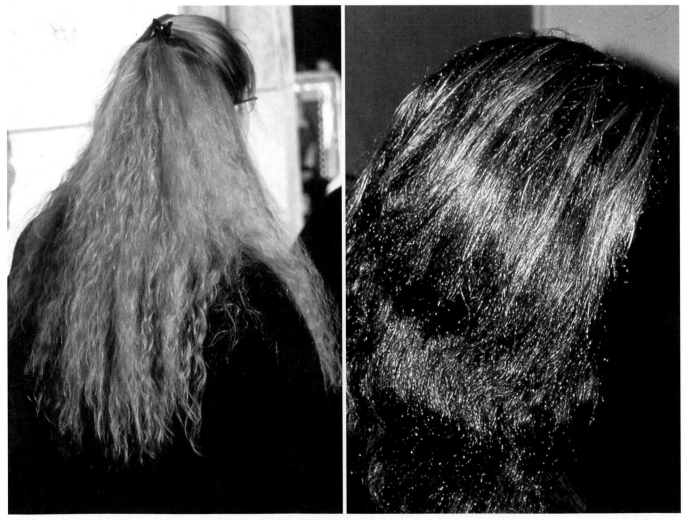

Damaged and porous hair may produce less than satisfactory results.

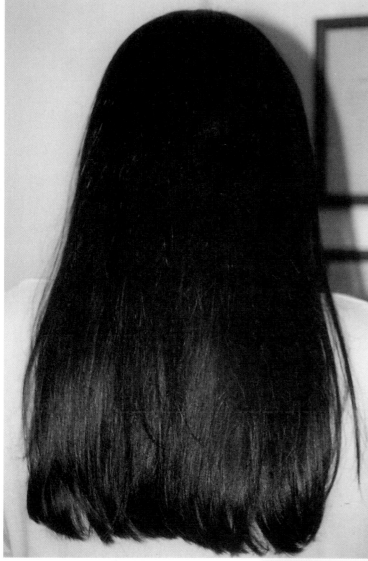

Oriental hair requires more dye than fine Nordic hair.

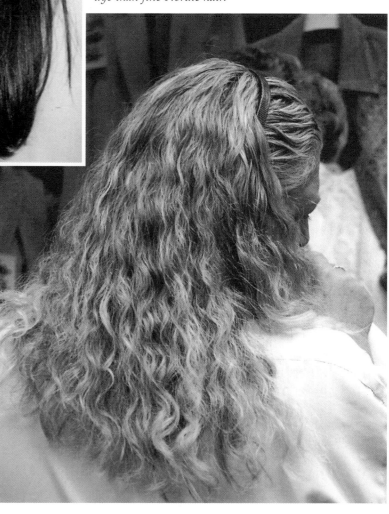

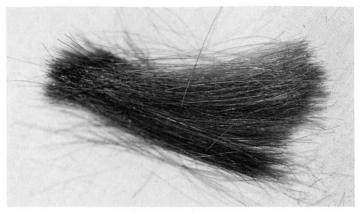

Always carry out a strand test to confirm the timing and anticipated shade result of your colouring.

■ In order to effect a change in naturally dark hair, the next step down is brown/red. To cover grey, stepping up to brown/black is the converse.

■ In considering how much we can effect a transformation the following chart reveals to what extent we can lighten (lift) dark brown hair – and why.

The shades seen on the product packaging may not produce the desired result for all the above reasons. A preliminary test – the so-called **strand test** – on an isolated portion of the hair is always advised.

Skin tone and eye colour

Always keep in mind your natural skin tone, as you want to choose a shade to complement your skin:

■ **Cool:** For skin that is olive, rosy brown, fair or rosy and eyes that are hazel, blue, blue-grey or green, the names of complementary cool shades will usually include the word 'ash'.

■ **Warm:** For skin that is fair to medium-golden, golden brown or darker and eyes that are deep brown, hazel or brown, the names of complementary warm shades will usually include the words 'warm', 'gold' or 'red'.

THE STRAND TEST

Do the strand test *each* time you colour to determine the timing and colour results. Permanent wave treatments, relaxers, previous colour and the sun can affect results and timing.

1. Cut a one-inch strand from the darkest or greyest part of your hair close to the scalp, and tape it at the cut end.

2. Completely cover the strand with the mixture remaining from the skin sensitivity test (see page 112). Start timing.

3. After 15 minutes, check the strand. If the strand is not the colour you want, return it to the mixture and check the colour every few minutes for up to 25 minutes.

4. For extra light blonding, more intense colour results or to cover resistant greys, it may be necessary to leave the hair colour on for up to 45 minutes.

HINTS AND TIPS FOR COLOURING HAIR

■ **Always read the instructions.**

■ Always complete a skin sensitivity test and a strand test before you begin colouring your hair, even if you have used the product before (see below).

■ If your hair is longer than shoulder length, or if it is very thick, you may need two boxes of colour to thoroughly cover all your hair with colour.

■ Follow the in-pack instructions carefully, paying particular attention to the development times. Use a timer so that the colour development timing is accurate, and start timing immediately after completing your hair colour application – not before.

■ Use a top-class shampoo and conditioner to keep your colour vibrant and your hair looking healthy and full of shine (see page 93).

Classical palette

A classical palette of colours could include:

Brunettes

Rich Burgundy Brown
Rich Lightest Golden Brown
Rich Light Golden Brown
Rich Light Brown
Rich Medium Golden Brown
Rich Bronze Brown
Rich Medium Brown
Rich Dark Brown

Reds

Radiant Light Auburn
Radiant Medium Red
Radiant Medium Auburn
Radiant Light Burgundy
Radiant Dark Auburn
Radiant Dark Red
Radiant Burgundy
Deeply Intense Copper
Deeply Intense Ruby
Deeply Intense Burgundy
Shimmering Deepest Burgundy

Blondes

Bleach Blonde Kit
Brilliant Extra Lightest Blonde
Brilliant Lightest Blonde
Brilliant Pale Cool Blonde
Crushed Pearl
Brilliant Light Golden Blonde
Brilliant Light Blonde
Brilliant Medium Golden Blonde
Brilliant Medium Blonde
Beige Shimmer
Brilliant Dark Blonde

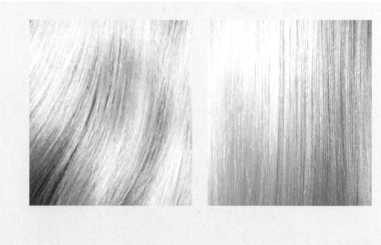

Step-by-step colouring

In this section we outline the actual process of permanent hair colouring.

Permanent dye products are sold as two components: one contains the dye precursors and ammonia in an alkaline base, while the second is a stabilized solution of hydrogen peroxide. The colours of the two may bear no relationship to the colour ultimately produced on the hair.

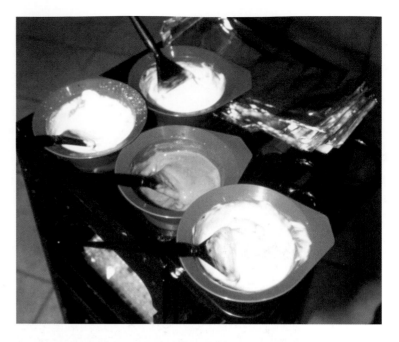

Permanent dye products are sold as two components, the colour base and the activator (hydrogen peroxide). Here we see more than one shade for professional applications.

Before

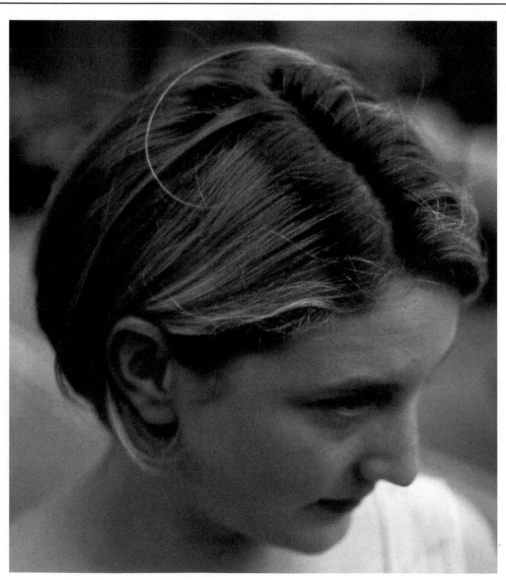

Step 1

The two components are mixed immediately prior to use, when the pH rises to almost 10. Again, the colour of this mixture may look nothing like the desired result.

Step 2

The mixture is applied to the hair, and the treated hair is wrapped in foil. Foil keeps the segments apart and allows different shades to be applied. It encourages penetration of the components into the hair shaft.

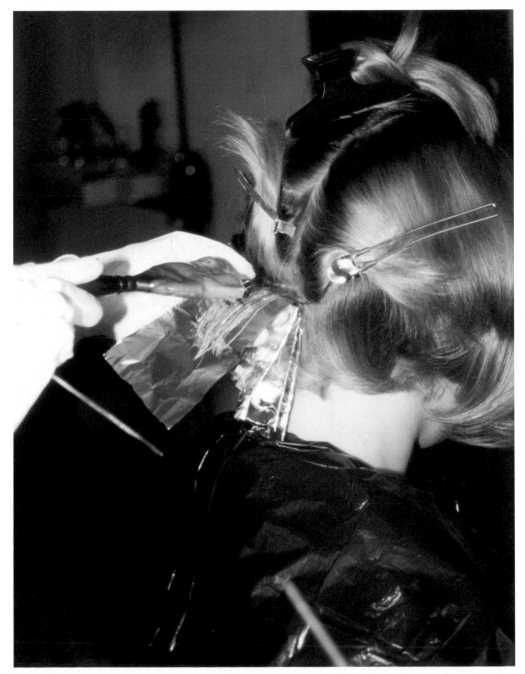

The mixture is applied to the hair.

Step 3

At high pH, the molecules of the dye precursors and peroxide diffuse into the hair shaft and react rapidly to form high-molecular-weight coloured materials.

The 'on-head' colour may look nothing like the shade selected, but it is vital *not* to wash off at this stage until the final colour is formed *inside* the hair. Rinsing too early may lead to a different colour altogether.

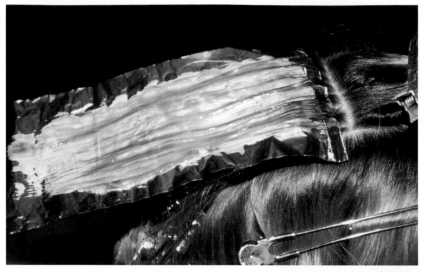

The 'on-head' colour may look bizarre.

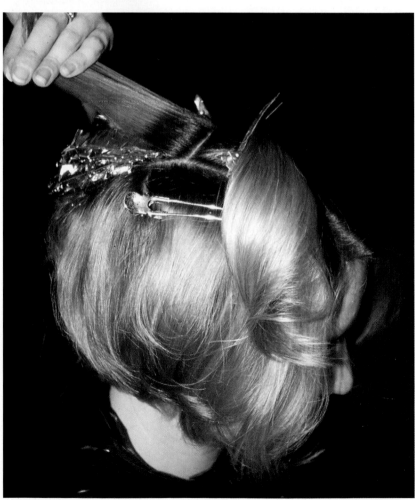

Colours are applied in segments.

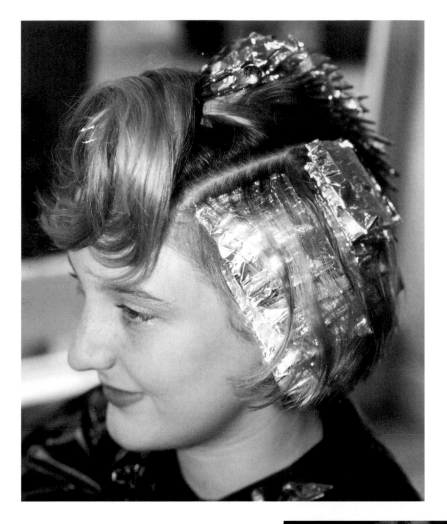

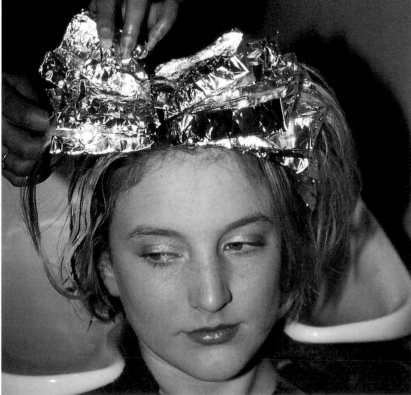

Colours are applied in segments

Step 4

After the time specified, rinse thoroughly and then apply the conditioner provided.

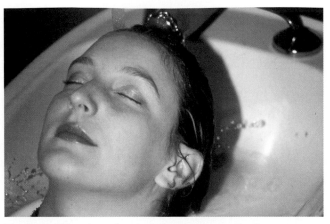

Time carefully, rinse thoroughly and then apply the conditioner provided.

Step 5

The end result, after careful drying and styling.

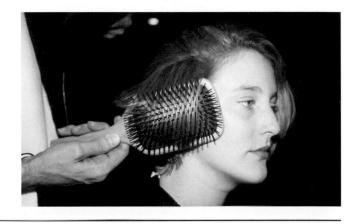

The end result!

Glamorous, subtle shades.

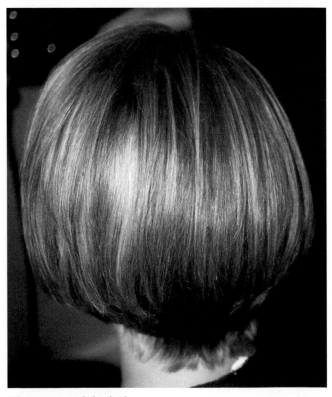

Glamorous, subtle shades

Roots

The problem with any hair dye is that it does not reach the newly formed hair in the follicle, and as hair grows approximately 1 cm a month the original natural colour (or lack of it) appears at 'the roots'.

Reapplication of colour to the roots is required to maintain the overall look. Excessive reapplication along the whole length of the shaft may result in excessive denaturing of protein, as a result of the bleaching action of the peroxide and its effect on the hair protein, keratin.

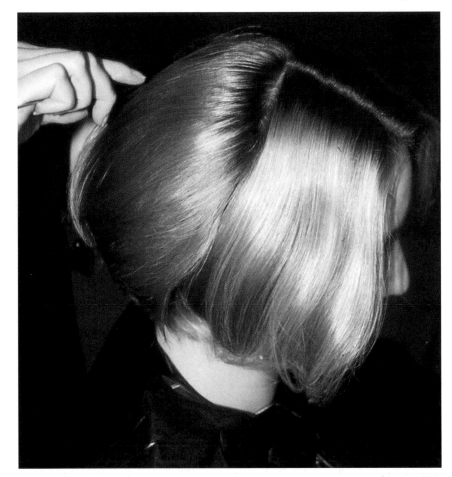

Attending to the roots.

SCIENCE BOX

Dye penetration of the hair shaft

Understanding how molecules penetrate the hair fibre is important for the cosmetic chemist.

Dye uptake, fastness, cosmetic ingredient penetration and final effect are all affected by this process. Recent work has led to greater understanding of the route into (and out of) the hair, and has led to better control of the movement of molecules from a formulation into the cortex of the fibre.

Within one or two minutes after immersion in solutions of water-soluble reagents, reagent molecules can be detected in all the structures of the hair shaft. They can be identified within the cuticle cell membrane complex (cmc) and the bulk of the cuticle cell at the same time, indicating different but complementary pathways into the hair fibre. There is evidence for pathways from the cmc into the bulk of the cuticle cell along the whole of the hair fibre.

The pigment does not wash out of the hair but remains within the core of the shaft. The lightening effect is due to an alteration in the light-absorbing properties of the melanin such that red light is reflected into the eye.

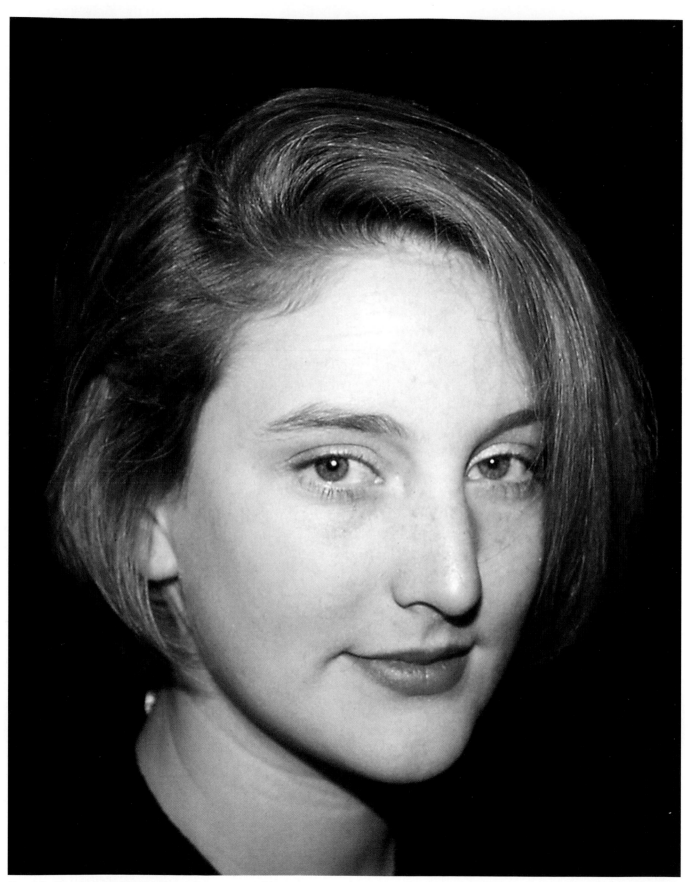

Four shades of professional colour enhance natural beauty.

Tips from the experts

Going blonde

Blondeness is a worldwide phenomenon in the 21st century. Around the world millions of women are going blonde. It is the single commonest hair salon procedure.

Going blonde (technically, 'lifting' the hair) is the result of the action of the peroxide on the pre-existing colour of the hair (due to melanin plus any residual dye). This 'bleaching' action allows the hair to be lightened and can also be important for grey coverage, where the bleaching brings pigmented and grey hair closer together in colour terms. Minimizing the colour difference between the hair types means that they move to similar final colours.

A note on semantics

'Up' (or 'Lift') refers to lightening the hair.

'Down' is adding a darker shade – for which covering grey hair is the commonest single reason.

SCIENCE BOX

- Bleaching is negligible below approximately pH 8, and increases significantly from pH 8.4 to pH 9.6.
- Key actives in bleaching are the peroxy anion (HOO^-) and ammonia (molecular ammonia, NH_3, not ammonium ion, NH_4^+), both of which predominate at high pH due to their pK_a values.
- Scalp irritation can occur with a high pH and a strongly buffered system. The measure of this combination of buffering and pH is termed the **reserve alkalinity** (RA).
- The harsher the conditions, the more hair damage is caused.
- Ammonia is almost universally used in high bleaching systems and in most medium and dark colours.
- Damage starts to occur as soon as the dye product comes in contact with the hair.
- Damage is caused by both radicals and peroxy anions.

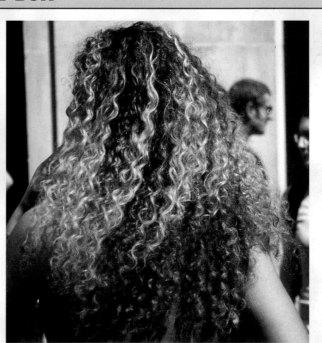

Hair damaged by over-treatment.

Practical steps in going blonde

A typical product marketed as, 'Blonde' provides a convenient method of lightening and toning, and will give maximum lightening of natural hair colour by a two-step process.

Step 1 – Blonde Lightener

Blonde Lightener is applied as a creamy gel, which will pre-lighten hair evenly in preparation for pale blonde toning. Products of this type may contain a blend of conditioners to protect the hair. Blonde Lightener is most effective when used on fair-to-brown hair.

Step 2 – Blonde Toner

This product is for use after lightening. The formula contains no ammonia or peroxide and has an easy-to-use shampoo-in formula. It can be used as a refresher between lightening applications.

A typical range might include Platinum Blonde, Warm Beige Blonde, Silver Blonde, Light Ash Blonde and Natural Pale Blonde.

Blonde highlights

A highlights kit allows the user to carry out blonde highlighting at home. A specially designed cap method or salon foil technique allows personalized highlights. An intensive after-conditioner is invariably included.

Such products are recommended for use on fair to medium-brown hair.

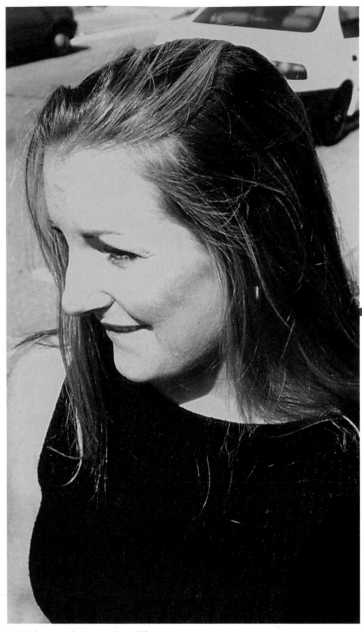

Mid-brown hair needs a lift.

Hints and tips for blonding your hair

- Follow the instructions carefully and always complete a sensitivity test and a strand test (page 84) before beginning blonding the hair, even if you have used the product before.

- Wear the gloves provided throughout the blonding process.

- Don't worry if red, gold or orange appears after the treatment begins. Most hair has to go through these stages before it arrives at blonde. Do *not* stop lightening, but continue until the mixture has been on the hair for the correct length of time, as indicated by the strand test.

- After blonding, use the intensive conditioner provided.

- Blonde Toner effectively tones pre-lightened hair, giving subtle shades of blonde.

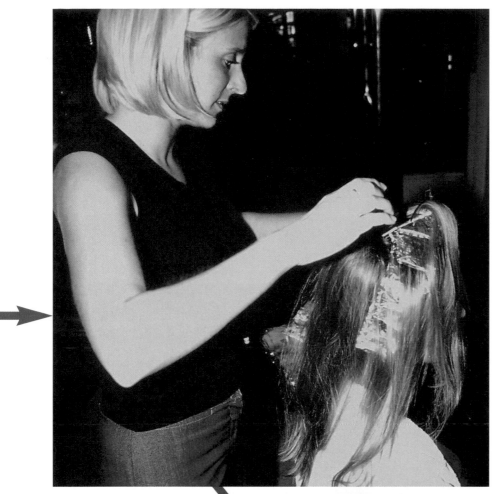

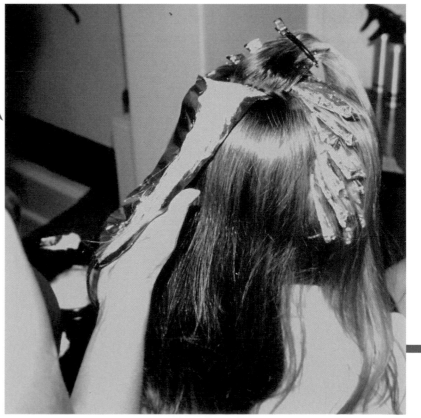

*Salon expertise in applying a
product. Oxidative chemistry
removes natural pigment and
supplies light tints.*

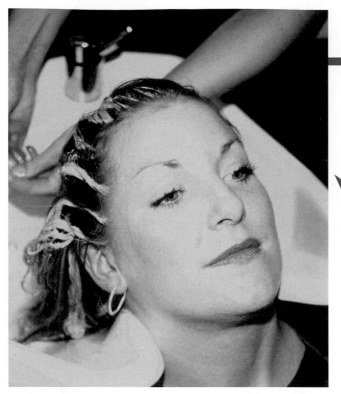

Rinsing thoroughly.

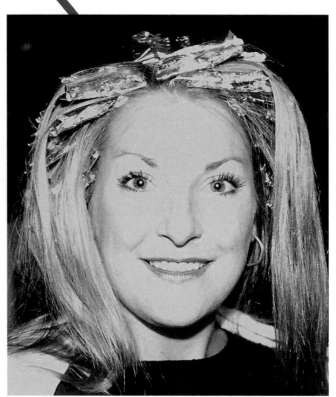

Getting the timing right.

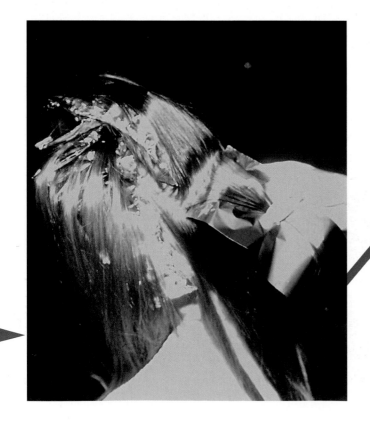

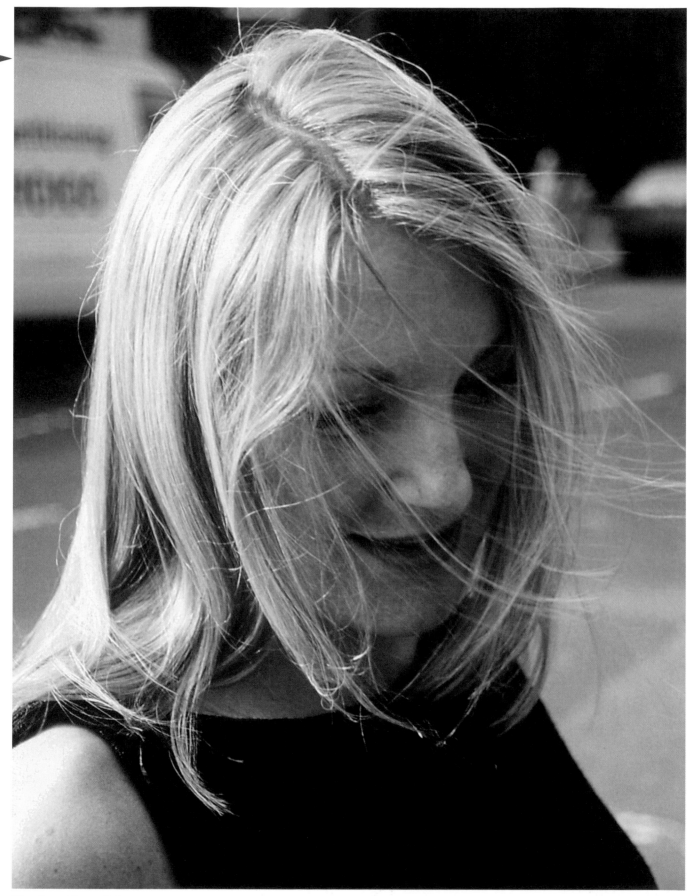

Blonde and beautiful.

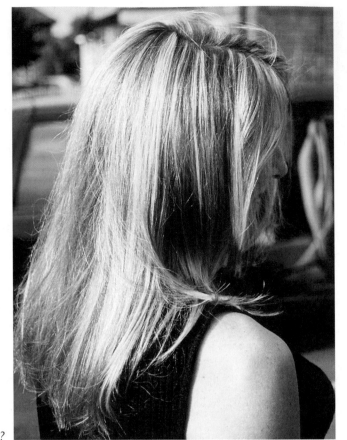

Time for a re-touch?

Hints and tips for highlighting your hair

- For subtle highlights, pull fine strands of hair through every other marked hole in the highlighting cap.

- For a more dramatic effect, use all the holes available in the highlighting cap.

- For a more natural look, highlight a few strands of hair on the crown (top) of the head.

- It may be helpful if a second individual helps to highlight the hair – two pairs of hands are sometimes better than one!

- If highlights need refreshing after a few weeks, remember that toners give new dimensions to highlights. Choose from different blonde shades, formulated without ammonia or peroxide.

Blonde Lighteners

If your natural starting hair colour is blonde to medium brown:
Blonde Lighteners are designed to allow those with naturally fair to medium-brown hair to achieve a very pale blonde effect. A strand test (page 84) performed before you begin will determine the development time required. Remember that naturally darker hair will take much longer to lighten to blonde.

- As hair is lightened, it will pass through several different stages from red to orange to gold to yellow. If your hair appears either red or orange this means that it has been insufficiently lightened and it will be necessary to leave the mixture on the hair and continue the development process.

- If the lightening mixture has been removed too early it is possible to repeat the application (allow a waiting period of 48 hours first), but you should pay attention to the condition of both the hair and the scalp. Over-processing can cause hair to become porous.

- If you have left the lightening mixture on the hair for the maximum recommended development time of two hours and you are still not satisfied with the degree of lightening, then the natural hair colour is too dark and further application is not recommended.

- Consult a salon for further guidance.

ITALY

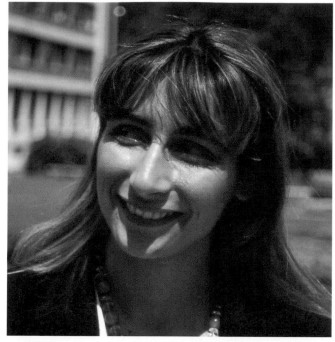

LONDON

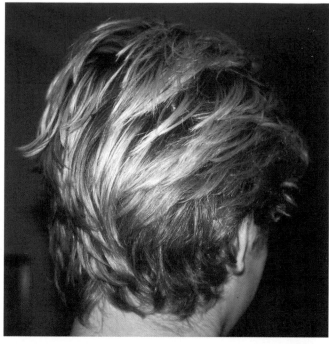

LONDON

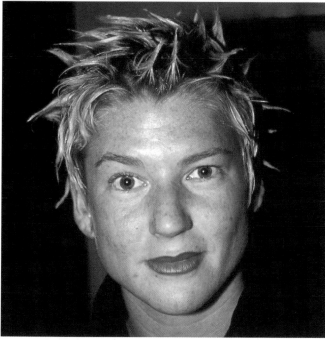

HONG KONG

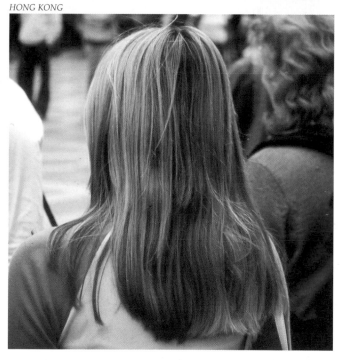

If your natural starting hair colour is dark-brown to black:
If your hair is naturally dark-brown to black, it may not be possible for you to become a pale blonde. A strand test will indicate how light your hair can go. The natural red undertones in hair may make it impossible to achieve a really light colour. If a Blonde Lightener has been used for the maximum recommended time and has not achieved the blonde result desired, a second application is not advisable. Visit the hairdresser, who will be able to suggest the best course of action to take.

If your starting hair colour is already blonde:
Blonde Toners add non-permanent colour to achieve a pastel shade.

If your hair has been lightened and you wish to return to the natural colour, visit a hairdresser who will be able to advise on re-pigmentation.

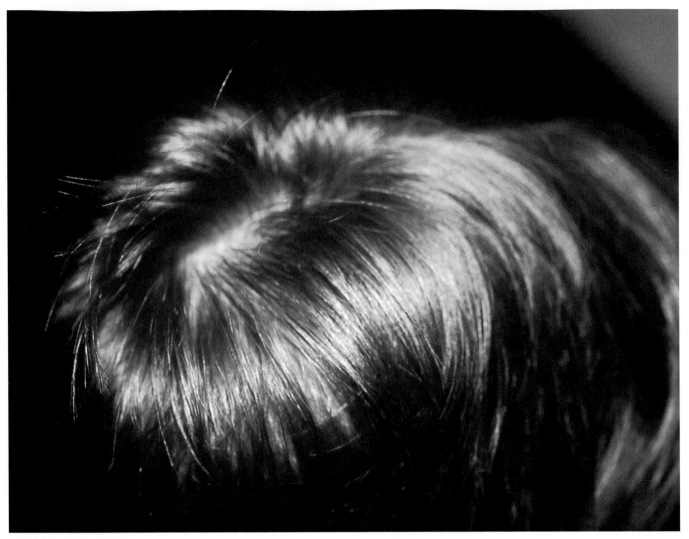

Red – The professional way.

Going red

Going red is popular worldwide.

Hints and tips for red shades

- The lighter your natural hair colour, the more vibrant the red shade will be.
- On high percentages of grey, some red shades may appear too vibrant and unnatural in appearance.
- In either of the above cases, the strand test will indicate the colour result.
- Red shades benefit from re-touches every 3–4 weeks to keep the colour looking fresh and vibrant.
- For maximum red intensity and longest-lasting colour results, always allow maximum development time.

Going brunette

Hints and tips for brunettes

- For the most natural looking results, select a shade within one or two shades of your own hair colour.
- Remember skin tone: selecting a shade much darker than your natural hair colour may look unflattering against a paler skin tone.
- If you wish to achieve maximum grey coverage, don't choose a shade more than one shade lighter than your natural hair colour.

Covering the grey

Covering the grey is the single most common reason for using hair dye products. There are three approaches to covering grey hair:

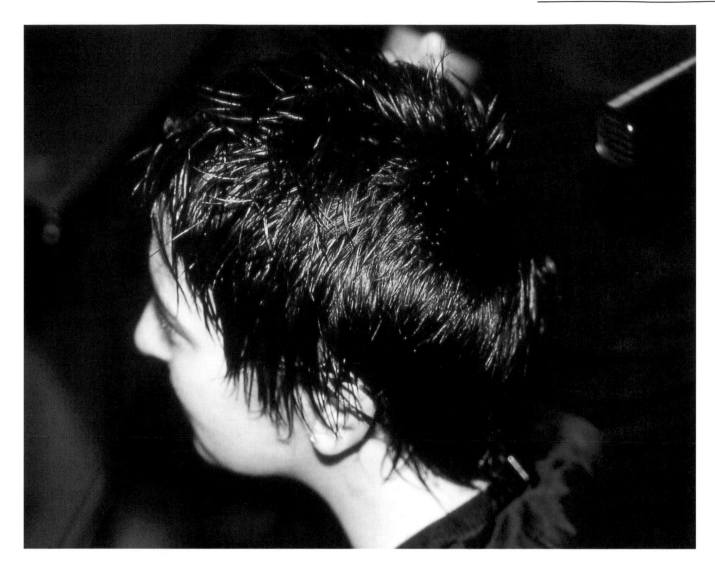

- to blend away grey and enrich one's natural colour
- to cover grey to match one's natural colour
- to cover grey while changing one's colour.

Choose Level 1, 2 or 3 colours to blend in or cover grey to match natural colour. Choose Level 3 colours to cover grey completely or change the natural hair colour.

To blend the first grey hairs into natural colour:
Use a hair colour close to the natural shade. Natural colour will look richer, shinier, and your few grey hairs will be covered to match. As long as grey is less than 50%, the grey will softly colour, and blend with overall colour.

A Level 1 colour that lasts for 6–8 shampoos can be used on the first signs of grey and where the grey is evenly distributed throughout the hair. If extensive grey is present (up to 100%), or there are concentrated patches of grey, a non-permanent Level 2 colour, which lasts through 24 shampoos, or a Level 3 permanent colour may be useful.

As the percentage of grey hair increases, select a shade slightly lighter than your natural colour, which will then blend and highlight the grey. With an increasing proportion of grey hair, skin tones tend to become paler too so a lighter rather than a darker hair colour is generally more flattering.

Covering grey either to match natural colour or to change it completely:
Cover grey completely with a permanent hair colour. Match your natural colour or darken, enhance or slightly lighten it. Level 3 permanent colorants are all suitable for this purpose.

Always check the pack to ensure the shade chosen is recommended for use on grey hair. For most effective grey coverage do not use a shade that is more than one shade lighter than your natural hair colour.

Tips for covering resistant grey hair

Resistant grey means that it is more difficult to cover the grey hairs, as more colour deposit is required to blend or match the grey to natural colour. A higher Level is needed to achieve better coverage. For example, to achieve 100% grey coverage you may need to move up from a Level 1 colorant to a Level 2.

Whether you are using a Level 1, 2 or 3 colorant, the following suggestions will help you get the best results:

- Leave the product on for the maximum time recommended in the product instructions. A strand test will determine how long a development time is needed to completely cover the grey.

- Deeper and darker shades cover grey better than lighter shades. Although Level 2 and 3 shades are all designed to cover grey effectively, the darker colours will achieve coverage more easily.

- Pre-soften the resistant grey areas first. For Level 2 and 3 colours, mix together one teaspoon each of colour and developer in a saucer (use a plastic teaspoon). Be sure to re-seal the bottles or tubes. Apply this mixture to resistant grey areas and time for ten minutes. Then mix the remaining colour and developer as normal and apply as usual to your hair. Ensure that the colour mixture is re-applied to the grey areas and leave on for the full development time before removing. For Level 1 colours, where no mixing is required, apply the colour directly from the bottle but follow the same procedure as for Level 2 and 3.

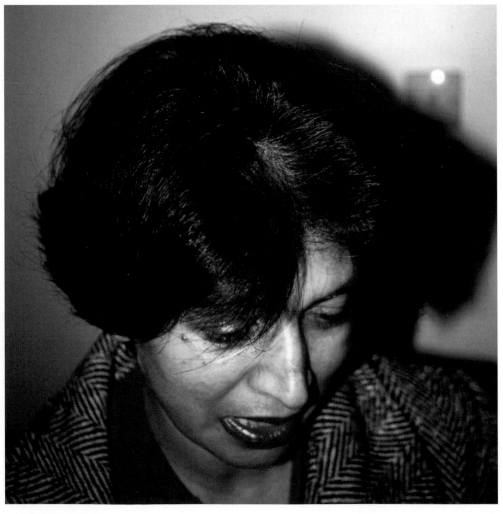

The single most common reason to colour – covering grey.

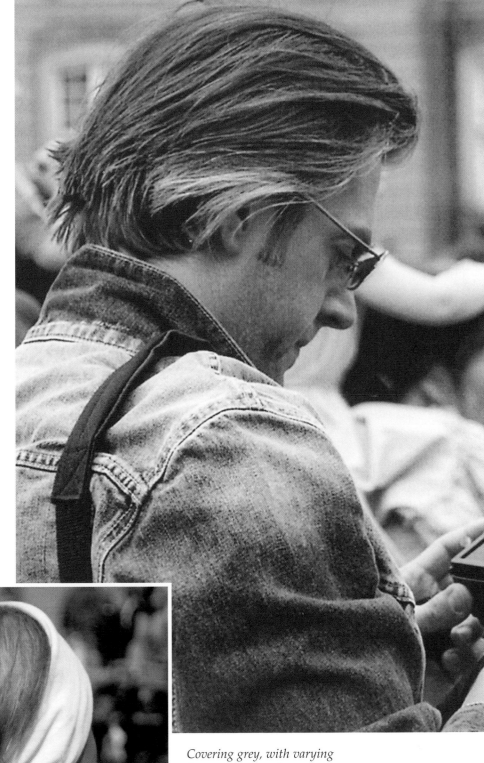

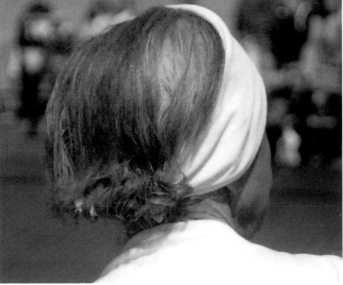

Covering grey, with varying
degrees of success!

Caring for your colour

Always use a shampoo and conditioner specifically designed for colour-treated hair, to ensure long-lasting colour and shine.

Repeated and/or excessive colouring can damage the hair by disruption of the protein in the cortex as well as the cuticle. So-called metal damage from copper present in some products or water sources is now known to be relevant.

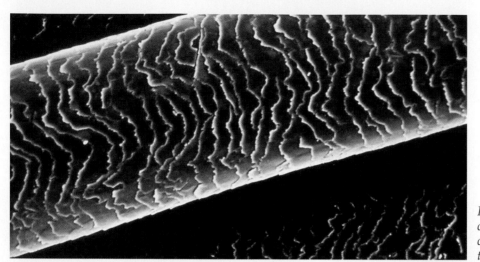

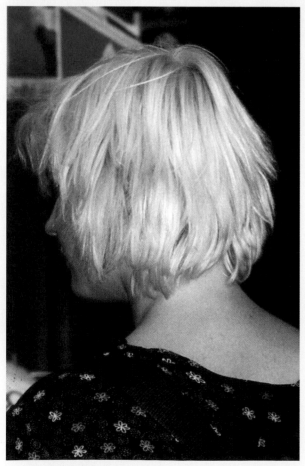

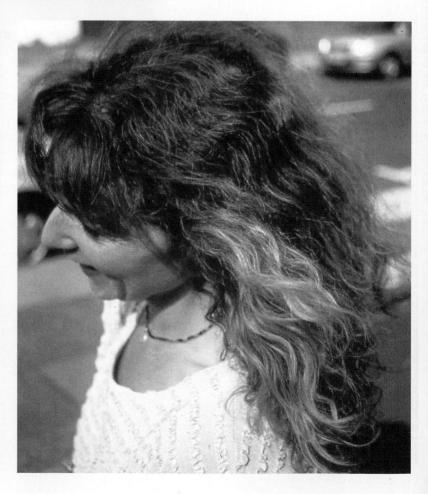

Repeated or excessive chemistry on the hair can lead to damage to the cuticle.

Repeated bleaching.

Colour problems

If all goes well, colouring hair can be life-transforming. As you will have realized by now, however, this apparently simple procedure is based on highly reactive chemicals. The cosmetic industry has striven to make it reliable but there may be occasions when the result falls short of the expectation. For example, the wrong shade may be the result of gross overambition, excessively processed hair or simply not reading the instructions.

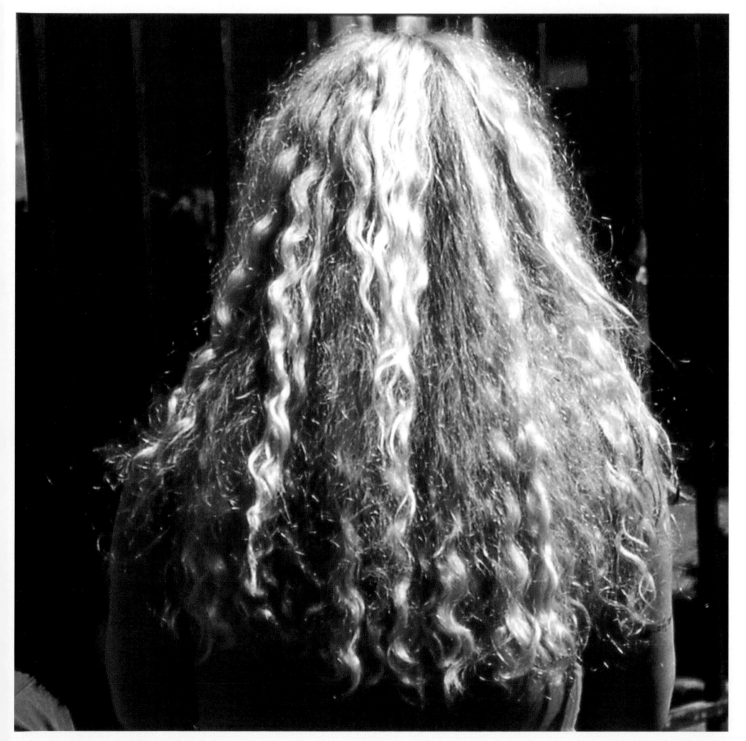

Colouring hair can be life transforming.

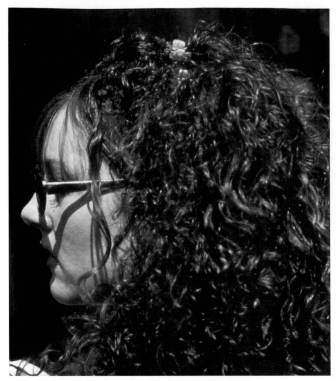

Unwanted reddish tones spoil the finished look.

In this section we look at some of the things that can go wrong and how to avoid them.

Orange, red or brassy tones?

Where hair has developed unwanted tones this is usually due to the use of a colour that is not appropriate for the natural hair colour. Another possible reason is that the hair is especially porous, or that there is a high percentage of grey hair.

The red/yellow tones that can be seen as melanin is bleached are undesirable and often termed brassy. They are now believed to be due to disaggregation of the oligomers.

How to remove unwanted warm tones:

■ Try using a similar shade containing ash tones to help tone down the unwanted warm colours (allow at least 48 hours between applications of permanent Level 3 hair colours).

■ Always remember to do a sensitivity test as well as a strand test, as described in the instruction leaflet.

The resultant colour may appear darker but should effectively eliminate the unwanted tone.

If, after performing the strand test, the colour is not acceptable do not proceed with the full application. Visit a hairdresser who will be able to remove the colour for you.

How to avoid unwanted warm tones:

■ Ensure that you buy the appropriate product for your natural hair colour. For example, a product designed to lighten fair hair will give a yellow or orange effect when used on dark-brown hair. Use the colour photographs on the back of the box as a guide only (each individual's hair is different) and remember that they represent the effect on natural hair, not on pre-lightened or coloured hair.

■ Always carry out a strand test (page 84 – you can do this at the same time as you perform your sensitivity test). This will give you an indication of the colour you can expect. If you are not entirely happy with this do not proceed. Instead, consider a more suitable shade or book a session with your hairdresser. You can always maintain the colour yourself at home.

■ Leave the colour to develop for the time recommended, or as indicated by the strand test. If you remove the product too quickly an orange tint can be produced because the product hasn't had enough time to either lighten your hair or to develop the colour fully. Do not use the colour of the mixture on the hair as an indication of the final hair colour result.

■ If your hair is especially long or thick, you may need to use more than one pack to achieve an even result.

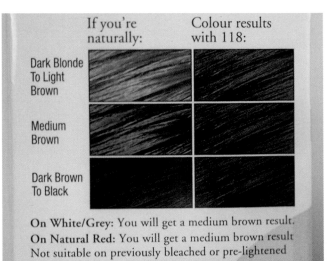

On pack colour guide.

■ If your hair is more than 15% grey or has concentrated patches of grey, you may find that you need to use a Level 2 product or a permanent colour. Always check the pack to ensure the shade is recommended for use on grey hair.

Unwanted purple tones in the hair

Experience has shown that where hair has developed an unwanted purple tone the reason is usually either that the hair is particularly porous or that there is a high percentage of grey hair. Either of these can result in uneven and unusual shades appearing as some of the dyes that make up the overall colour are absorbed more quickly than others. The outcome can be seen as purple tones in the hair.

How to remove these tones:
If you have used a shade that is much darker than your hair's natural colour, it may take some time for the colour to be removed completely. You can speed up the process by washing your hair more frequently. Using a hot oil treatment and wrapping your hair in a warm towel will also help the colour to wash out more quickly.

How to avoid these tones in the future:
The appearance of purple tones usually indicates that it is time to upgrade to a higher Level product to achieve better grey coverage. Move up from a Level 1 to a Level 2 product, or use a Level 3 product (permanent) to achieve the best 100% grey coverage.

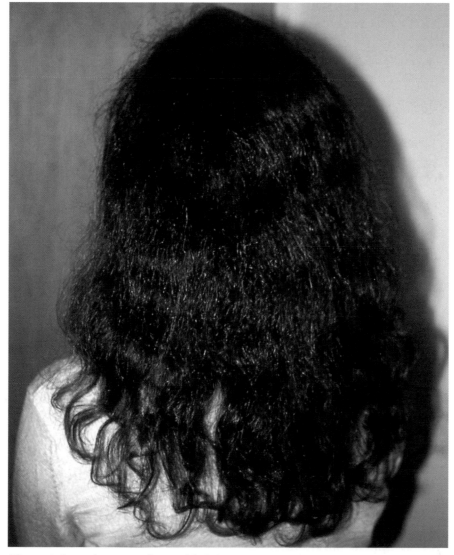

Unwanted purple tones – damaged hair is a common cause.

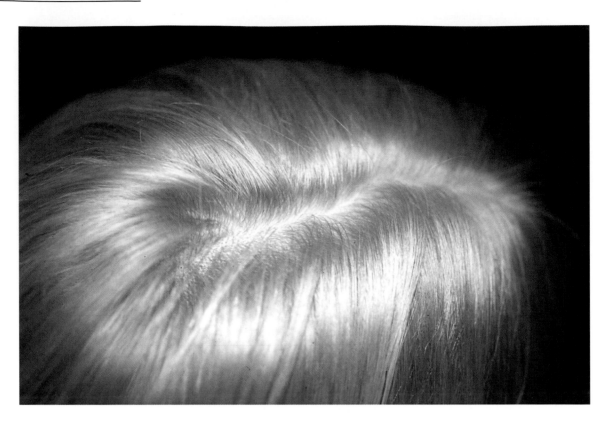

Problems with red hair

Fading colour

Whatever colour is employed, hair will look its best when the hair colour is fresh. Although reds are just as easy to create as any other hair colour, re-colouring is necessary more often to keep the red vibrant. This is because the red pigment molecules are small and tend to shampoo out or lighten more quickly than other hair colours.

Tips to help you keep your red vibrancy longer:

- Red shades benefit from re-touches every three or four weeks.

- If you are using a Level 3 permanent red, use a Level 1 colour to keep the colour looking fresh (use a similar shade).

- Use a shampoo and conditioner especially formulated for colour-treated hair.

- Condition your hair every time you wash it, as conditioners make hair less porous.

- Use a weekly deep-conditioning treatment or a leave-in conditioner for all-day moisturizing and protection if your hair is very long, thick, dry, damaged, or frizzy.

- Ensure you allow the maximum development time as suggested in the instruction leaflet.

Hair colour 'coming out' during washing:

For the vibrant red shades it may be necessary to rinse hair for longer than normal to remove the colorant after the recommended development time. The rinse water should be running clear before you use the conditioner that is provided with the colorant.

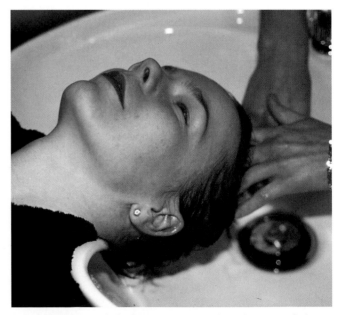

For the vibrant red shades you may need to rinse your hair with extra care.

Hair colour too dark?
Why does hair colour sometimes develop darker than expected? Experience has shown that the reasons why the result is too dark may be either:

- Hair is especially porous and is accepting colour more readily than normal. Porous hair can be caused by chemical and physical factors (perming, using heated appliances, swimming in chlorinated pools and strong sunlight). Over-application of Level 3 permanent colours may also increase the hair's porosity.

- The colour used was not appropriate for the natural hair colour.

- Colour product has been applied to already coloured hair, leading to a build-up of colour. For this reason the mid-lengths and ends may look darker than the roots.

- Permanent hair colours will not wash out, but grow out, although the colour will lighten slightly with time. If a blonde colorant has been used it may be possible to lighten it very slightly by using a paler blonde shade. If a light brown or darker colorant has been used, however, it may not be possible to lighten the resultant shade with any other product. A hairdresser may be able to remove the colour for you.

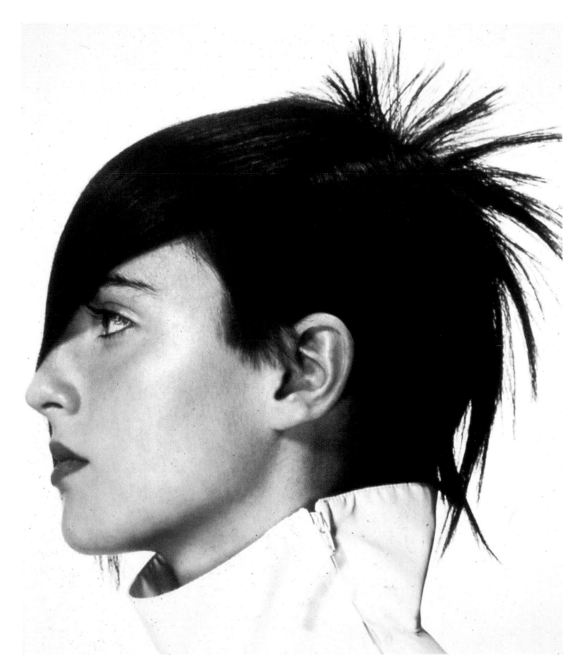

Permanent hair colours will not wash out (though they will grow out), but the colour will lighten slightly with time.

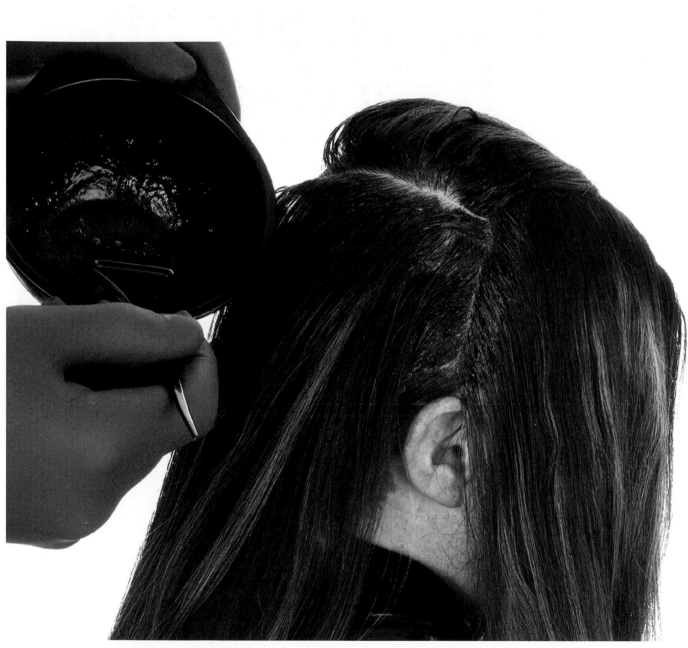

Hair dyes are potent chemicals – regulations cover health and safety for all who may come into contact with them.

[*Source* HABIA skills team]

8

The safety of hair dyes

PPD and its derivatives are still the most important molecules in the hair dye arena, particularly where darker shades are needed. They remain the most effective ingredient for permanent hair colouring, and as most of the world has dark hair and covering the grey is so frequent, the scale of human use and exposure over many decades has been truly significant.

In any debate regarding the safety of hair dyes, it must be remembered that every day *millions* of people, both women and men, employ these products without significant ill effects and with very considerable quality-of-life benefits.

PPD is a highly reactive molecule, and is able to link up with other chemicals to form long-chain molecules in the hair shaft, imbuing it with a new colour. Since it is very reactive (it is a hapten, an incomplete antibody stimulating substance) it does have the potential to combine with a protein molecule in the skin. In turn this may lead to sensitization (creation of antibodies by the immune system) and on future reapplication, an allergic reaction such as dermatitis with eczema may occur on the face or neck where product has been spilled. This may be a severe reaction, but an acute swelling like bee sting allergy is rather rare.

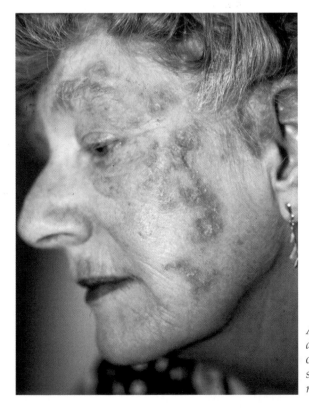

An allergic reaction such as dermatitis sometimes occurs; rarely, this may be severe or acute swelling, resembling bee sting allergy.

This unfortunate and often unpredictable phenomenon is recognized by both manufacturers and regulators. The estimated frequency of serious reactions is approximately one in a million applications, and these are more commonly experienced with products delivering very dark shades, in which the concentration of PPD is highest.

Manufacturers label their products with safety warnings to reduce the risk of allergic reaction. Following the directions on the duration of the skin test application is important. All good salons should follow this procedure and should not apply hair dyes without carrying out this test several days before the full appointment.

Whether the product is applied in the salon or at home, the person applying it *must* wear adequate gloves, and it is desirable that mechanical or cream barriers are used to prevent any spillage on to the skin. The hair is the main target for the hair dye and problems may occur where product has run directly on to the skin.

Despite all these precautions reactions can occur at any time after the first exposure. Cross-reaction with other similar dyes is known, and unregulated tattoos may expose the individual to PPD. In Europe PPD is prohibited for this purpose.

For years, the industry has hunted for an alternative to PPD. All those investigated so far have failed to come close to the depth and versatility of this precursor, and customers have rejected products that do not offer the quality of current dyes. Yet, curiously, many people with established allergy still persist in using permanent hair dyes despite advice as to the risk: such are the quality-of-life benefits they perceive.

THE SKIN ALLERGY TEST

Hair colour products may cause allergic reactions, which in rare instances can be serious.

Do not colour if you have had a previous reaction.

To help minimize your risk it is important to perform the skin allergy test 48 hours prior to every application.

1. Mix small equal parts of Hair Colour and the Colour Activating Crème in a plastic bowl.

2. Apply a small amount of the mixture to the inside of your elbow. Allow to dry. Do not wash this area for 48 hours. (Use the remaining mixture for your strand test, see page 84.)

3. Examine the test area during the next 48 hours. If no reaction occurs, you are ready to colour.

4. If any rash, redness, burning or itching occurs you may have an allergy and you must *not* use this product.

It is important to follow this advice. Many people at home and even in salons may ignore it and proceed to colouring without testing.

Skin allergy reactions are very rare, however, relative to the numbers of people who colour every day and over many years without incident. But as with peanuts, penicillin and even the humble carrot, an allergy to this product or to one of its ingredients can occur.

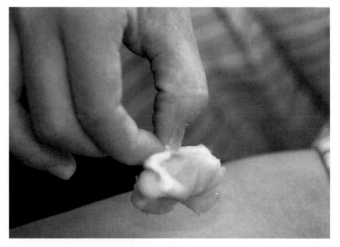

The skin test: applying the colour with cotton wool or cotton bud.

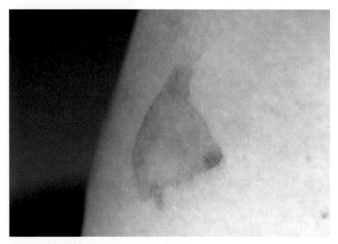

*Skin staining. If redness and swelling occur – do **not** proceed with colouring.*

Hair dye products are regulated in Europe, North America and Japan, and PPD and other ingredients are permitted under the various cosmetic directives in these regions.

Although no alternative to PPD has been discovered, the skill of the cosmetic formulator has allowed a marked reduction in concentration in products compared with a decade ago by increasing use of other molecules with which it can combine.

Fashion changes, disguising grey or simply a change at or after a 'life' event are now possible with safe and reliable products.

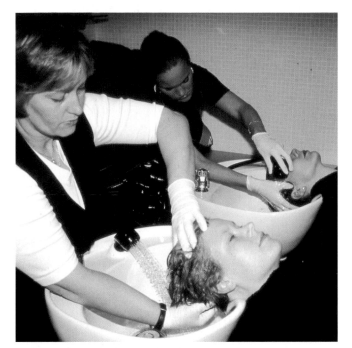

Gloves are essential during application and rinsing.

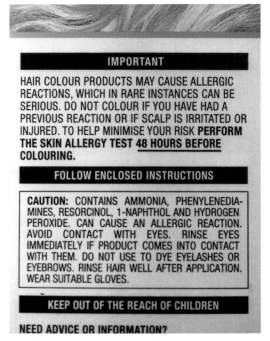

IMPORTANT

HAIR COLOUR PRODUCTS MAY CAUSE ALLERGIC REACTIONS, WHICH IN RARE INSTANCES CAN BE SERIOUS. DO NOT COLOUR IF YOU HAVE HAD A PREVIOUS REACTION OR IF SCALP IS IRRITATED OR INJURED. TO HELP MINIMISE YOUR RISK **PERFORM THE SKIN ALLERGY TEST 48 HOURS BEFORE COLOURING.**

FOLLOW ENCLOSED INSTRUCTIONS

CAUTION: CONTAINS AMMONIA, PHENYLENEDIA-MINES, RESORCINOL, 1-NAPHTHOL AND HYDROGEN PEROXIDE. CAN CAUSE AN ALLERGIC REACTION. AVOID CONTACT WITH EYES. RINSE EYES IMMEDIATELY IF PRODUCT COMES INTO CONTACT WITH THEM. DO NOT USE TO DYE EYELASHES OR EYEBROWS. RINSE HAIR WELL AFTER APPLICATION. WEAR SUITABLE GLOVES.

KEEP OUT OF THE REACH OF CHILDREN

NEED ADVICE OR INFORMATION?

Labelling of hair colour products: an example.

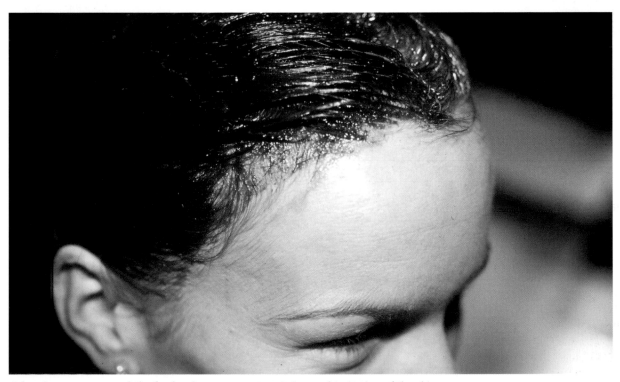

A barrier cream around the forehead may prevent staining and irritation of the skin.

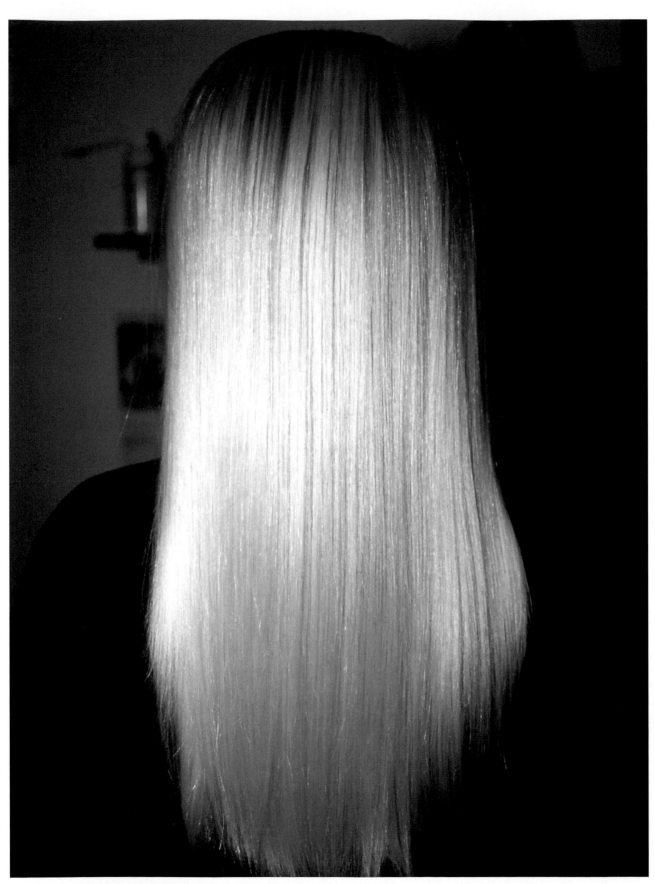

Fabulous blonde hair – the peak of achievement of both chemist and stylist.

9

Hair colour products: regulatory issues

The complexity of the chemistry and toxicology of hair colorants has been outlined in previous chapters. From a regulatory viewpoint hair colorants attract more attention than other cosmetic categories for two main reasons:

- the potential of some hair colorant ingredients such as *p*-phenylenediamine to cause allergies,
- the chemical reactivity of oxidative hair colorants and the fact that many dye precursors are arylamines (some of which are known to be harmful in certain circumstances).

Firstly, allergy potential is a well-known trait of hair colorants and it continues to be carefully monitored by the industry working with dermatologists.

Secondly, media attention periodically focuses on the potential of hair dyes to cause cancer, based on sometimes sensationalized and inaccurately interpreted scientific data. However, one needs to carefully follow up the scientific literature and to remain alert in case a problem would occur. Nevertheless, sophisticated tests based on a tier battery approach, including many different types of systems, have improved our knowledge in this area and provided clear evidence in support of the safe use of hair colorants. Large scale epidemiology studies actually did not demonstrate a clear association with any type of cancer even with life time use of hair colorants.

Much debate was triggered in the popular press by a 2001 study investigating an alleged association between bladder cancer and the use of hair colorants. Following this, the EU Scientific Committee for Cosmetics and Non-Food Products (SCCNFP, now superseded by the Scientific Committee for Consumer Products, SCCP) requested more data on hair colorants' potential genotoxity and eventual carcino-genicity. This is perhaps one of the reasons (but not the only reason) that precipitated a new regulatory review by the EU Commission. In the US, however, the Cosmetic Ingredient Review (CIR) decided to undertake a major review of all the epidemiology data available on hair colorants to date. A report analysing 83 epidemiological studies on hair colorants was submitted to the CIR Epidemiology Review Panel in August 2003, and the Panel's verdict was *'The authors found insufficient evidence to support a causal association between personal hair dye use and a variety of tumours and cancers.'*

Worldwide regulations

Hair products, particularly those using active chemistry (for example, hair colorants and permanent waving products), present important challenges to safety assessors and regulators worldwide. Products using complex chemistry are used by millions of consumers throughout the world, with a fairly simple regulatory approach based on robust safety assessments.

Hair products are regulated in most of the world as 'cosmetics'. Regulations in this area do not generally require strict pre-marketing approval controls in most developed countries, but the level of responsibility and liability that cosmetic safety assessments involve is often quite similar to that which applies to food and drug assessments.

European regulations

Hair products in the European Union and the European Economic Area are regulated by the Cosmetics Directive 76/768/EEC, of which Article 2 states that cosmetics must not cause any harm to the user under normal or foreseeable conditions of use, taking into account the instructions for use of the product.

Annex III to that same Cosmetics Directive constitutes a list of substances permitted under particular conditions and/or concentrations and includes several hair colorant precursors and couplers, e.g. paraphenylenediamine, aminophenols and resorcinol. Actually, all oxidative hair dyes are under study by the SCCNFP (future SCCP), based on toxicological dossiers provided by the companies concerned. The outcome of this important exercise will be the elimination of old substances and/or substances for which insufficient data are available, as well as the preparation of a positive list of hair dyes. All Annexes to the Cosmetics Directive are kept up to date by the ATP (Adaptation to Technological Progress) procedure which, through a relatively rapid system, maintains specific ingredient regulations. The advisory body to the EU Commission with regard to changes via the ATP procedure was, until July 2004 the Scientific Committee for Cosmetic Products and Non-Food Products intended for consumers (SCCNFP). It is now superseded by the Scientific Committee for Consumer Products (SCCP) a new committee with a similar mandate to the SCCNFP, namely to advise the EU Commission on all consumer products that are non food and non drug products. The responsibility for adapting the legislation, however, does not lie with the scientific committee, but entirely with DG Enterprise.

As already mentioned, actually hair colorants have to comply with Annex III listings for precursors, couplers and hydrogen peroxide and a set of specific labelling provisions especially designed for hair colorants. These labelling provisions address the allergenic potential of some ingredients such as p-phenylenediamine. Specifically Annex III requires the following labelling for p-phenylenediamine:

- Can cause an allergic reaction
- Contains p-phenylenediamine
- Do not use to dye eyelashes or eyebrows.

Finally, when developing new products, it is always important to consult Annex II of the Cosmetic Products Directive, since that particular Annex lists all the substances that are forbidden to being used in cosmetic products, thus also in hair dyes.

US regulations

The Food, Drugs and Cosmetics Act designates the Food and Drug Administration (FDA) as the regulatory body responsible for cosmetic safety. As in the EU, cosmetics may be marketed freely without any pre-marketing checks.

Cosmetic colour ingredients that are used for colouring hair are regulated in one of two ways. Firstly, there is a list of approved colours that may be used for colouring hair, and in other cosmetics such as eye-shadows. Only 36 FDA 'certified colours' and 23 'permitted colours' are on the approved colour list for use in cosmetics. Secondly, hair dyes that are derived from coal tar may be used to colour hair as long as the product is labelled with the following statement: 'Caution – This product contains ingredients which may cause skin irritation on certain individuals and a preliminary test according to the accompanying directions should first be made. This product must not be used for dyeing the eyelashes or eyebrows; to do so may cause blindness.' The accompanying package must provide directions for carrying out the sensitivity test.

The CIR (Cosmetic Ingredient Review) process is a mechanism set up by all interested parties to review cosmetic ingredients. The CIR panel in the US serves a similar function to that of the SCCP in the EU, although the regulatory systems to execute CIR and SCCP recommendations are different. There is no direct regulatory action following CIR reviews; however, CIR deliberations are regarded highly and usually reputable manufacturers comply with their

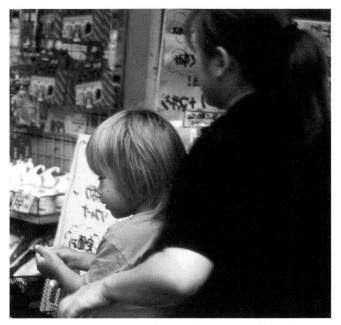

Manufacturers discourage the use of dyes on children's hair.

recommendations as if they had regulatory status. The CIR in the US and the SCCNFP in the EU often compare their deliberations and conclusions on ingredients.

Japanese regulations

All cosmetic ingredients in Japan have to be listed in a 'positive list', the CLS (Comprehensive Licensing Standards of Cosmetics by Category). Until 2002 all cosmetics also had to be authorized by the Ministry of Health and Welfare (MHW) before marketing. After 2002 the MHW granted a de-regulation for cosmetics and now only the listing in the CLS is sufficient to market cosmetics. However, many product categories considered cosmetics in the US and the EU are considered quasi-drugs in Japan. These are hair colorants, permanent waves, products to combat bad breath, bath preparations, talcum powder, depilatories, shaving lotions and some skin products. These still require pre-registration with the MHW. Japan is the only country in the developed world still working with a partial pre-registration system for cosmetics.

Some regulatory considerations for other countries

Many countries around the world are looking at the EU Cosmetics Directive as a model. In Latin America, for example, many countries have adopted a de-regulated system that is expected to embrace more and more the self-registration mechanism seen in the EU. Other countries like China have recently relaxed their cosmetics importation rules in line with European legislation, although hair colorants still require a cumbersome registration and ingredients have to be on a positive list.

Even the recent Japanese de-regulation is based on the EU 'self-registration' mechanism. This de-regulation trend will probably continue on the basis that cosmetics regulations in the EU and the US provide a strong level of consumer protection without the need for pre-market registration.

All regulations reviewed here can be considered simple when compared with those applying to pharmaceuticals. However, the post-market controls by authorities and the legal liability imposed on the manufacturers and their safety assessors are rigorous, and are generally considered to be sufficient. No major concerns around users' safety exist, and the key fundamentals of the 'self-registration' regulatory models employed in the US and the EU are being adopted more and more by other countries worldwide. Key recent examples in Japan, China and Latin America indicate that cosmetics regulations are moving towards a common direction. There is a good precedent in this very area of global harmonization: the International Nomenclature of Cosmetic Ingredients (INCI) is a virtually global language for cosmetic ingredients – no other consumer products can boast such an historic regulatory achievement. On this basis one can be optimistic and expect that eventually cosmetics will be self-regulated globally, perhaps with a set of harmonized rules that will allow total global exchange and consumer-safe circulation of these products.

And finally…

We hope you have enjoyed this book. If and when you decide to make that transformation, remember that hair dye products offer glorious opportunities for your quality of life. However – **do please read the instructions**.

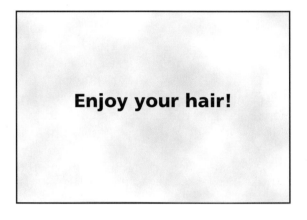

Index

Page numbers in *italics* refer to illustrations or captions only.

achromotrichia 35
active intermediates *67, 69*
additive colour mixing 15
agouti signalling protein (ASP) 45
albino people 10
alkalizing agents 64, 70
allergic reactions 111–12, 115
amelanotic melanocytes 32
ammonia, alkalizer 70, 93
ammonium persulphate, alkalizer 70
anaemia 35
anagen 22
Andamanese people 10
ASP *see* agouti signalling protein

black/dark hair *10, 20,* 22, 23, *36, 38,* 43, 75–6, *83*
   bleaching *42,* 43
   changing hair colour to 100
   curly *7, 8, 10, 18, 20, 23, 38*
   dominant in humans 5, *37,* 43
bleached hair *5, 30, 42, 66, 71*
   in history 53–5
   light reflectance 28, *29*
bleaching *see* blonding hair
blonde hair *4, 7, 11, 20,* 22, *38,* 43, 46–9, *50, 54,* 76, *83, 114*
   children's *19, 20, 23, 26, 38,* 47
   in maturity 48, *49*
   whether gentlemen prefer 77
   see also bleached hair
Blonde Lighteners 94, 98
Blonde Toners 94, 99
blonding hair 53–4, 93–7
blue hair 35
bonobos 8
brassy tones 106–7
brightness 16

cancer
   risk from hair colorants 115
   skin 8,

canities *see* grey hair
catagen 22
chelants 70–71
children's hair *19, 20, 22, 23, 26, 27, 46, 47*
   use of colorants discouraged 117
chroma 16, 17
CIE La*b* colour system 17
circle of colour *15*
Clairol hair colorants 55, 56
colour blindness 16
colour couplers *67, 68, 69*
colour developers *68, 69*
colour in nature 3–4
colour perception 12–16
colour precursors *67, 68, 69*
colour systems 17
colour terminology 16–17
cone cells 12–13, *14, 15,* 16
cortex of hair 67
couplers *see* colour couplers
curly hair *10, 18, 23, 27, 38, 66, 74, 93, 105*
cuticle of hair *67, 104*

damaged hair *30,* 82, 93, 104
damaged skin 8,
dendrites 21
dietary deficiencies 35
dopaquinone *19, 24, 25*

early humans 4, 8, 10, 47
eumelanin *19, 25,* 26, 43, 45
European regulation of hair colour products 115, 116, 117
eye 13–14

fatty alcohols, in hair colorants 71

genetic factors 10
   colour vision 12
   hair colour 7, 37, 43–4, 46

golden hair 40
green hair 35
grey hair 26, 27, 30–35, 82
    covering 32, 34, 72, 76, 93, 100–102, 103, 107
    resistant 102

hair
    function 8, 10
    structure 67
hair bulb 21
    of shed hair 22
hair colorants 51–79
    choosing a shade 77, 81–4
    classical palette 85
    depths and tones 77
    development 57–61
    historical background 53–6
    natural and vegetable 78–9
    penetration of hair shaft 91
    problems in using 105–9
    regulations 115–17
    safety issues 111–13
    see also permanent hair colorants; semi-
    permanent hair colorants; temporary hair
    colorants
hair colour 4–5, 7–12, 28–35
    caring for 104
    evolution 8–10, 43
    fantasizing about 76, 77
    in history 37–49
    pigments 19–27, 29
    psychological aspects of changing 72–6
    stereotyping 41, 48, 75–6
hair cycle 22
hair dyes see hair colorants
hair follicle 19
hair patterns 12
henna 53, 54, 78–9
highlights xiv, 4, 6, 34, 42, 76, 94, 98
hue 16, 17
hydrogen peroxide 64, 67, 69, 70, 72

INCI (International Nomenclature of Cosmetic
    Ingredients) 117
iodopsin 14

Japan, regulation of hair colour products 117

keratinocytes 21
kidney disease 35
kwashiorkor 35

labelling of hair colorants 112, 116
lanugo hair 26
LCH colour system 17
Level 1 colorants 64
Level 2 colorants 64, 65
Level 3 colorants 64, 65
light refraction 13
lightening hair see blonding hair
lightness 17

MC1R see melanocortin 1 receptor (MC1R)
medulla of hair 67
melanins 7, 21–2, 24–5
    see also eumelanin; phaeomelanin
melanocortin 1 receptor (MC1R) 24, 44, 45
melanocyte-stimulating hormone (MSH) 24
melanocytes 21–2, 33
    amelanotic 32
melanosomes 21–2, 24
migration of humans 8–10, 37, 45
MSH see melanocyte-stimulating hormone
mummy
    blonde-haired 47
    with dyed hair 53

nature, colour in 3–4
nephrotic syndrome 35

opponent theory of vision 14
oxidative chemistry (colorants) 62, 69, 95

permanent hair colorants 55, 56, 64–5, 67–72
    application 86–90
    packaging 61, 77, 113
    problems with 109
phaeomelanin 19, 25, 26, 37, 43
    resistance to bleaching 28
p-phenylenediamine (PPD) 55, 67, 111, 112, 113,
    116
photoprotective function of hair 8,
porous hair 109
PPD see p-phenylenediamine
precursors see colour precursors
primary colours 15
    psychological 16
primates 4, 5, 8
purple tones 107

red hair vii, xvi, 10, 20, 23, 37, 39–40, 43–5, 48, 57,
    72, 76
    artificial 50, 78, 79, 100
    light reflectance 28
    problems with 108

reflectance of hair 28, *29*
   measuring *61*
refraction of light 13
regulation of hair colour products 115–17
reserve alkalinity 93
retina *13*, 14, 16
rhodopsin 14
rod cells 14, 16
roots, reapplication of colour 91

safety
   in laboratory *60*
   in use of colorants 111–13
saturation (colour) 16
semi-permanent hair colorants *63*, 64
signalling 8, 12
skin allergy test 112
skin damage 8,
skin pigmentation 10
skin tone 82
smoking
   and grey hair 33, 35
   and hair colour 35
social implications of hair colour 37, 39
solvents, in hair colorants 71

strand test 84
substrate 64
sunlight 3
surfactants, in hair colorants 71

telogen 22
temporary hair colorants 62
thermoregulatory function of hair 8

uniforms 37, *39*
unwanted tones in coloured hair 106–7
USA, regulation of hair colour products 115, 116–17

virgin hair, light reflectance 28
visual purple *see* rhodopsin
vitamin A 14
vitamin D 47

weathering 29–30
Wella hair colorants *55*, 56
white hair 5, *27*, 28, *31*

yellow hair 35